CARDIOLOGY RESEARCH AND CLIN

HEAT SHOCK PROTEINS IN CARDIOVASCULAR DISEASES

CARDIOLOGY RESEARCH AND CLINICAL DEVELOPMENTS

Additional books in this series can be found on Nova's website
under the Series tab.

Additional E-books in this series can be found on Nova's website
under the E-books tab.

PROTEIN SCIENCE AND ENGINEERING

Additional books in this series can be found on Nova's website
under the Series tab.

Additional E-books in this series can be found on Nova's website
under the E-books tab.

CARDIOLOGY RESEARCH AND CLINICAL DEVELOPMENTS

HEAT SHOCK PROTEINS IN CARDIOVASCULAR DISEASES

SATORU TAKEUCHI
J. GERALDINE SANDANA MALA

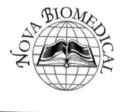

Nova Science Publishers, Inc.

New York

NOTICE TO THE READER

The Publisher has taken reasonable care in the preparation of this book, but makes no expressed or implied warranty of any kind and assumes no responsibility for any errors or omissions. No liability is assumed for incidental or consequential damages in connection with or arising out of information contained in this book. The Publisher shall not be liable for any special, consequential, or exemplary damages resulting, in whole or in part, from the readers' use of, or reliance upon, this material. Any parts of this book based on government reports are so indicated and copyright is claimed for those parts to the extent applicable to compilations of such works.

Independent verification should be sought for any data, advice or recommendations contained in this book. In addition, no responsibility is assumed by the publisher for any injury and/or damage to persons or property arising from any methods, products, instructions, ideas or otherwise contained in this publication.

This publication is designed to provide accurate and authoritative information with regard to the subject matter covered herein. It is sold with the clear understanding that the Publisher is not engaged in rendering legal or any other professional services. If legal or any other expert assistance is required, the services of a competent person should be sought. FROM A DECLARATION OF PARTICIPANTS JOINTLY ADOPTED BY A COMMITTEE OF THE AMERICAN BAR ASSOCIATION AND A COMMITTEE OF PUBLISHERS.

Additional color graphics may be available in the e-book version of this book.

Library of Congress Cataloging-in-Publication Data

Takeuchi, Satoru.
Heat shock proteins in cardiovascular diseases / Satoru Takeuchi, J. Geraldine Sandana Mala.
p. ; cm.
Includes bibliographical references and index.
ISBN 978-1-61324-589-7 (softcover)
1. Cardiovascular system--Diseases. 2. Heat shock proteins. I. Mala, J. Geraldine Sandana. II. Title.
[DNLM: 1. Cardiovascular Diseases--pathology. 2. Heat-Shock Proteins--therapeutic use. QU 55.6]
RC667.T35 2011
616.1'06--dc23
2011014538

Published by Nova Science Publishers, Inc. † New York

Contents

Preface

The cardiovascular system is a prone target to stress and other genetic and physiological perturbations that need to reduce the severity of the pathological progressions. Cardiovascular diseases (CVD) are on the rise since the past decades and recently awareness of the CVDs has been proved to be vigilant amongst the modern population. Hence, a deeper insight into the various CVDs and the protective HSP responses is necessitated. *Heat Shock Proteins in Cardiovascular Diseases* provides a keen insight into the various abnormalities of the human heart and the upregulation of the heat shock proteins in cardiovascular stress. Description of the many heart ailments that are prevalent with notes on their aetiology and pathogenesis are specifically discussed with essential information on the induction of heat shock proteins in response to cardiac stress, its physiological roles and prospects of using the heat shock proteins in therapeutics. A correlation of the fundamental roles of HSPs in cardiac pathological conditions is elaborately discussed. The protective potentials of HSPs could be essential to salvage cardiac tissues during repetitive cardiac stress and limit disease progression. Therefore, it is attempted to evaluate the stress response of the predominant HSPs in cardiovascular dysfunctions and enumerate their potencies to combat the stress overload and restore normalcy. An understanding of the novel properties of the HSPs as potential candidates for therapeutics is concluded in a separate section.

The proposed book is intended for Research and Professional reference purposes. The principal audience of this book is aimed towards all researchers working on heat shock proteins, medical doctors specializing in cardiovascular abnormalities and the general research community wanting to pursue in heat shock proteins in cardiac diseases. This book would be handy for research students in their research profession.

Acknowledgments

The authors gratefully acknowledge the financial support of Mr. Kikuji Takeuchi and Mr.Naomi Takeuchi of Takenen, Japan.

Dr. J. Geraldine Sandana Mala wishes to sincerely thank Dr. Satoru Takeuchi, Presidentof Takenen, Japan, for his constant encouragement and support in rendering the completion ofthis book. She also expresses her deep sense of gratitude to her parents, Mr. A.J. JohnBromeo and Mrs. Helen Bromeo, sister, Ms.J.Rita Jasmine Ranjani, for their deep affection and moral support towardsthe preparation of this book, to her brothers, J.Maria Thomas and J.Justin Arul Xavier, sister-in-law, Mrs. Sundari Thomas, nephew, Master John Bala and niece, Little Priya. Illustrations provided byMs. J. Rita Jasmine Ranjani are gratefully acknowledged.

In: Heat Shock Proteins …
Authors: S. Takeuchi and J. G. S. Mala

ISBN: 978-1-61324-589-7
© 2012 Nova Science Publishers, Inc.

Chapter I

Introduction

Abstract

From discovery to the diverse array of cellular functions, heat shock proteins represent one of the groups of highly specialized proteins that maintain cellular homeostasis, monitor protein folding during metabolic stress and aid in prevention of apoptotic mechanisms. Designated according to their molecular mass, heat shock proteins are upregulated and manifested upon stress and act to mend the protein conformational stability during protein unfolding and prevent protein aggregation.

Due to chaperoning effects, heat shock proteins are also referred as molecular chaperones in respect of their profound abilities in rendering correctly folded proteins after protein translation in the cytosol. This book is therefore dedicated to the unique class of heat shock proteins especially, mammalian proteins in their identities and responses in the cardiovascular system.

1.1. Heat Shock Proteins – The Discovery

Early in the 1960s, an accidental incubation of *Drosophila* at an elevated temperature in a Genetics laboratory in Italy led to observations of puffed chromosomes that were later identified as an increased activity of heat shock genes. In 1974, the concept of heat shock proteins (HSPs) was established during cellular stress and heat shock treatments. This upregulation of an array of proteins in response to stress was the first step towards global research of the ubiquitous group of proteins that associate and perform a challenging role in protein folding both constitutively, and mostly upon induction. Heat shock proteins exhibit evolutionary conservation and occur from bacteria to humans. Consequently, HSPs have been known to display chaperoning roles during protein folding and are termed as molecular chaperones of the cell.

Since then, extensive research of these molecules have resulted in the identification of their roles in ER-associated and cytosolic protein folding, refolding during stress, prevention of protein aggregation due to protein misfolding, intracellular protein trafficking, anti-inflammatory and antioxidative effects, inhibition of apoptosis and other cellular events that highly contribute towards maintenance of the stress overload and restore cellular normalcy.

HSPs are represented according to their molecular mass and thereby classified as HSP110, 90, 70, 60 and small heat shock protein families. Another classification is based on their cellular localization and therefore grouped as Endoplasmic reticulum (ER) chaperones and cytosolic members and also mitochondrial stress proteins. The ER chaperones are usually constitutive in basal amounts sufficient for chaperoning functions.

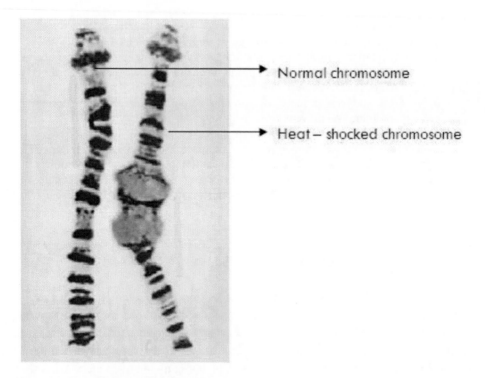

Normal chromosome

Heat – shocked chromosome

Figure 1.1. Heat shocked puffed chromosome.

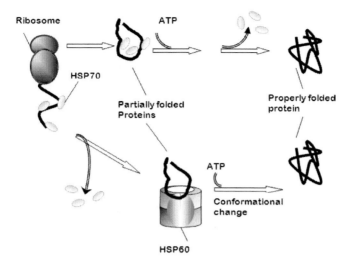

Figure 1.2. Molecular chaperones in concerted protein folding.

Production of high levels of heat shock proteins can also be triggered by exposure to different kinds of environmental and pathophysiologicalstress conditions, such as UV irradiation, toxicity of arsenic and trace metals,infection, inflammation, exercise, exposure of the cell to toxins, starvation, hypoxia or water deprivationand their upregulation is described more generally as part of the stress response.

Table 1.1. Protective roles of heat shock proteins

HSP family	Major functions	Clinical Manifestations
HSP110	Protein disaggregation, thermotolerance	Hypoxia; heat; osmotic stress
HSP90	Regulatory interactions with signaling proteins, stabilization of misfolded proteins	Heat stress; ischemia; hypoxia; oxygen radicals; proinflammatory cytokines
HSP70	Protein folding, membrane transport of proteins	I/R injury; heat stress
HSP60	Protein folding (limited substrates in eukaryotic cytoplasm)	Ischemia; heat stress
Small HSP	Stabilization of misfolded proteins, thermotolerance, eye lens structural proteins	I/R injury; apoptosis; Dox-induced cardiac dysfunction

1.2. Phylogeny and Homology

HSPs are structurally and functionally well-conserved stress proteins. HSP110 family has been classified based on phylogenetic analysis. Amino acid and nucleotide sequences were aligned using CLUSTAL-W 1.83. A phylogenetic tree was constructed using the NJ (neighbor-joining) algorithm.The mammalian HSP110 family member sequences were retrieved from GenBank. Accession numbers of the sequences: human HSC70 (protein, P11142; mRNA, NM_006597), dog HSC70 (protein, XP_536543; mRNA, XM_536543), rat HSC70 (protein, XP_001053026; mRNA, XM_001053026), mouse HSC70 (protein, NP_112442; mRNA, NM_031165), human GRP78 (protein, NP_005338; mRNA, NM_005347), dog GRP78 (protein, XP_537847; mRNA, XM_537847), rat GRP78 (protein, NP_037215; mRNA, NM_013083), mouse GRP78 (protein, NP_071705; mRNA, NM_022310), human HSP70RY (protein, BAA75062; mRNA, AB023420), dog HSP70RY (protein, XP_861723; mRNA, XM_856630), rat HSP70RY (protein, NP_705893; mRNA, NM_153629), mouse HSP70RY (protein, NP_032326; mRNA, NM_008300), human HSPA4L (protein, ABM69040; mRNA, EF197155), dog HSPA4L (protein, XP_533297; mRNA, XM_533297), rat HSPA4L (protein, XP_215549; mRNA, XM_215549), mouse HSPA4L (protein, NP_035150; mRNA, NM_011020), human HSP110 (protein, BAA34779; mRNA, AB003333), dog HSP110 (protein, XP_534515; mRNA, XM_534515), rat HSP110 (protein, NP_001011901; mRNA, XM_213699), mouse HSP110 (protein, NP_038587; mRNA, NM_013559), human ORP150 (protein, ABC75106; mRNA, DQ350134), dog ORP150 (protein, XP_536547; mRNA, XM_536547), rat ORP150 (protein, NP_620222; mRNA, NM_138867),. and mouse ORP150 (protein, NP_067370; mRNA, NM_021395). ER members of GRP78 and ORP150 and the cytoplasmic members of HSC70, HSP70RY, HSPA4L, and HSP110 have been classified based on the phylogenetic tree obtained.

OSP94 belongs to the HSP110 subfamily because of its homology to HSP110 (65% identical) and HSP70RY (62% identical) by homologous sequence search. Inspite of its homology to most heat shock proteins by BLASTX, BLASTP search failed to identify similar sequence homology due to non-conserved regions within the C-terminal half of OSP94, which showed sequences of divergence (Val^{497}-Gln^{594} and Lys^{707}-Asp^{838}). This prompted us to investigate the sequence homology and similarity patterns in the class of mammalian OSP94 proteins.

Consensus sequences were observed with most sequences by CLUSTAL W indicating this highly conserved class of mammalian stress protein (Mala and Takeuchi, 2009).

Evolutionary changes might have contributed to a lower degree of non-homologous sequence patterns, which is however of bare significance amongst the mammalian HSP110 family. OSP94 is also observed to exhibit partial similarity with an 105 kDa molecular chaperone with 24 amino acid residues.

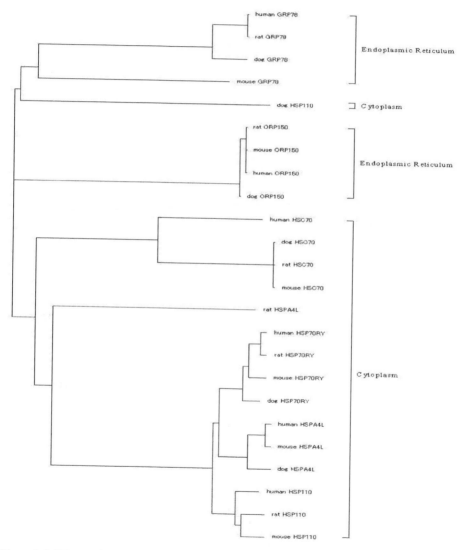

Figure 1.3. NJ tree of HSP110 members.

1.3. Er Chaperones in Protein Folding

Translated polypeptides need to attain three-dimensional structure for their biological activities. The process of protein folding ensures correctly folded conformations of the proteins assisted by several chaper ones and folding catalysts. Protein folding in the ER lumenmust occur in high concentrations of nascentpolypeptide chains and at a high concentration of total protein, which increase the aggregating behavior of the folding proteins. Molecular chaper ones act by preventing unproductive intra- and inter-molecular interactions, enabling the unfolded polypeptide to reach the defined structure specified by its amino acid sequence. The newly synthesized polypeptides therefore fold in hierarchically ordered chaper one pathways.

Molecular chaper ones are among themost highly expressed proteins in the cell. The ER resident chaper one BiP/GRP78 accounts for 3% of the soluble protein content of the cell, while, all chaper ones and folding enzymes together contribute to 15-25%. The chaper ones and folding enzymes interact with one another in large complexes and form a dense network-like structure within the ER lumen. Chaper ones belonging to HSP70 and HSP60 families cooper ate in cellular pathwaysof protein folding. HSP70s function primarily in prevention of premature misfolding of nascentpolypeptides, while, HSP60 family mediate the folding of moltenglobule-like intermediates to the native state. Critical steps of folding and rearrangement occur in the shielded environment of the chaper one cavity. Protein folding is fundamental to cellular processes and inspite of the abundance of the folding machinery, protein misfolding and protein aggregation due to cellular stress form the basis of many pathological conditions and disease mechanisms.

1.4. Ischemic Preconditioning

The heart possesses a remarkable ability to adapt itself against any stressful situation by increasing resistance to adverse consequences. This phenomenon, known as 'ischemic preconditioning', is an inherent ability of the myocardium to protect itself from ischemic damage. Ischemic preconditioning is the manifestation of earlier stress response that occurs during repeated episodes of brief ischemia and reperfusion, and can render the myocardium more tolerant to subsequent lethal ischemic injury. This adaptive protection was first described by Murry and collaborators in 1986 and has been found to be mediated by gene expression and transcriptional regulation. Preconditioning involves a cascade of stress signals such as activation of protein kinase C(PKC), protein tyrosine kinases(PTKs) and mitogen-activated protein kinases(MAPKs). These kinase modulations effect the opening of K_{ATP} channels, expression of a number of protective proteins known as heat shock proteins (HSPs), upregulation of nitric oxide synthase(NOS), induction of cyclooxygenase-2 (COX-2)and cellular antioxidants. In humans, ischemic preconditioning has been shown to occur in patients undergoing coronary angioplasty with significantly less STsegment deviation, lower mean pulmonary artery pressure, lower cardiac vein flow and less myocardial lactate production during the second balloon inflation. Acute MI with antecedent angina patients have a lower mortality, a small infarct size and a lower incidence of complications than patients whose acute MI was not preceded by angina. The early form of ischemic preconditioning, referred to as, 'classic' preconditioning is observed immediately following brief sublethal ischemia and conferred a marked slowing of the progression of ischemic injury during subsequent ischemia. A distinctive feature of classic preconditioning is that the protection afforded by antecedent ischemia rapidly lapses out. In most subjective models, no protection against infarction was observed if the preconditioning and the subsequent ischemic insult extended beyond 2 h period and is therefore, short-lived. A delayed form of adaptation is manifested subacutely around 24 h following preconditioning with ischemia, variably known as, 'delayed' preconditioning; 'late' preconditioning; 'second window' preconditioning or 'second window of protection' and is observed as a protection against a variety of ischemic pathologies.

1.5. Hsp-Mediated Cardioprotection

Currie and co-workers introduced the concept of heat stress preconditioning as a strategy for myocardial infarction in 1988. It was therefore proposed that heat stress preconditioning was beneficial for the ischemic myocardium. Preinduction of HSP70 protected cardiovascular function following trauma-hemorrhage and resustication. Between 1995-1996, it was demonstrated that overexpression of HSP70 protected the heart against the damaging effects of ischemia using a variety of determinants such as infarct size, creatine kinase release, recovery of high energy phosphate stores and correction of metabolic acidosis. The cardioprotective mechanisms of HSPs involve the inhibition of mitochondrial caspase 9 pathway of apoptosis by HSP27, HSP90 and HSP70. HSP27 can protect the integrity of the microtubules and actin cytoskeleton in cardiac myocytes and endothelial cells exposed to ischemia.

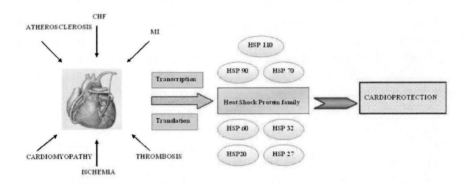

Figure 1.4. Cardioprotection of heat shock proteins in stress.

Also, HSP90 has been shown to bind to endothelial nitric oxide synthase and stimulate its activity. Further, the overexpression of HSP70 enhanced NO production in response to cytokine stimulation. HSP70 has also been identified as a cytoprotective therapeutic agent which decreases the risk of postoperative atrial fibrillation by reducing I/R injury. Mild-to-moderate alcohol consumption is also associated with an induction of the expression of several cardioprotective proteins such as heat shock and antioxidant enzymes.

Of recent interest, Kwon et al. in 2007 have analyzed the efficiency of protein transduction domain (PTD)-mediated delivery of HSP27 on I/R injury. This represents a potential therapeutic strategy as protein drug for ischemic heart diseases. Free radicals formed by oxidative stress in myocardial I/R injury, result in ventriculardysfunction, or "myocardial stunning," arrhythmias, andprogressive cell damage or death after ischemic injury. Molecular chaperones effect cardioprotection to counteract the reactive oxygen species (ROS) by mediating the protective roles of glutathione peroxidase (GPx), superoxide dismutase (SOD) and catalase.

References

Mala JGS and Takeuchi S (2008) Heat shock proteins in cardiovascular stress. *Clin.Med:Cardiol* 2: 245-256.

Mala JGS and Takeuchi S (2008) Molecular chaperones of mammalian ER in protein folding and quality control. In: *Heat shock proteins: New Research*, ed. Morel E and Vincent C, Nova Publishers, USA, pp.1-27.

Mala JGS and Takeuchi S (2009) Molecular cloning of OSP94: A significant biomarker protein of the human hypertensive heart and a member of HSP110 family. *Mol. Biotechnol.* 42:175-194.

Saitou N and Nei M (1987) The neighbor-joining method: a new method for reconstructing phylogenetic trees.*Mol. Biol .Evol.* 4: 406–425.

Thompson JD, Higgins DG and Gibson TJ (1994) CLUSTAL W: improving the sensitivity of progressive multiple sequence alignment through sequence weighting, position-specific gap penalties and weight matrix choice.*Nucleic Acids Res.* 22: 4673–4680.

In: Heat Shock Proteins …   ISBN: 978-1-61324-589-7
Authors: S. Takeuchi and J. G. S. Mala   © 2012 Nova Science Publishers, Inc.

Chapter II

Heat Shock Proteins

Abstract

Heat shock proteins are upregulated and manifested upon cellular stress and possess chaperoning functions. The molecular chaperones are essential guardian components of the cell and predominantly serve as the machinery in protein folding and quality control. The characteristic chaperones and their distinctive features contributed by structural domains are described. The mechanisms of heat shock protein expression and their subcellular localization are focused in this Chapter. Protein folding in the ER is elaborated to provide an insight into their primary chaperoning roles. A short note on inhibition of apoptosis is discussed which offers promising approaches of heat shock proteins in the near future.

2.1. Molecular Chaperones

Heat shock proteins (HSPs), originally named due to their induction upon heat stress are structurally and functionally well-conserved class of stress proteins and found in all organisms from bacteria to humans. Heat stress leads to a number of cellular events such as protein denaturation, transient cell cycle arrest, changes in membrane fluidity and increased turnover of plasma membrane proteins. HSPs serve to offer cellular adaptation and enhanced protection that is rapidly effected to tide over the stress overload. HSPs constitute important family characteristics that contribute to their chaperoning functions. The primary function of HSPs is to regulate protein folding by functioning as intracellular chaperones in protein interactions and assist in precise folding to attain proper protein conformations.

Normally, the chaperone function is to assist in the protein folding after posttranslational modifications encountered in the ER which are then secreted in their native conformations essential for cellular activities. They are upregulated under stress and act to prevent unwanted protein aggregation and help to stabilize partially unfolded proteins and their transport across the cell membrane. HSPs function to aid quality control by proteasomal degradation of misfolded/malfolded proteins that cannot be used by the cell in extreme stress. An important feature of heat shock proteins is their evolutionary conservation from bacteria to the mammalian species exhibiting homology patterns among their protein sequences. The sequence patterns are not only similar, but also are the stress response and expression patterns suggesting critical functions in cellular adaptation.

HSPs are triggered by a variety of cellular stress stimuli and are pronouncedly induced while under normal physiological conditions, they are synthesized in basal amounts. The marked increase in their inducible expression is regulated by the heat shock protein transcription factor HSF which is phosphorylated into its active trimers that associate with the heat shock element HSE and result in the transcription of the HSP mRNA. In addition to protein folding, HSPs display antioxidant effects, aid protein refolding, protect membranes from damage and inhibit apoptosis. Recently, HSPs are also known to bind cell-surface receptors and exhibit immunomodulatory functions. Non receptor-mediated uptake of HSPs has also been identified consequently in antigen presentation that has implications in immunoregulatory mechanisms. Loss-of-function of HSPs compromises their ability to handle stress while gain-of-function promotes cellular protection. We describe the major classes of HSPs that perform characteristic functions and grouped according to their molecular mass.

2.1.1. HSP110

A major HSP family belongs to the HSP110 class that possesses chaperoning functions to assist in appropriate protein folding. The HSP110 class proteins are distant relations of the HSP70 class and comprise of GRP78, HSP110, ORP150, HSP70RY and OSP94.

HSP110

HSP110 has been recognized as a major heat shock protein since the past two decades especially in the mammalian cells. HSP110 family is known to be distinct from the HSP70 family differing in its molecular mass as well as by a sequence divergence from the archetypical HSP70s. HSP110 also shares some related functions as that of the HSP70 and has been shown to confer cellular heat resistance and prevent protein aggregation and maintain denatured proteins in a folding-competent state. The chaperoning functions of HSP110 have been described with identification of functional domains by use of targeted deletions. This study summarizes essential points on its structural data (i) the ATP-binding domain is functional, but appears to be normally masked, (ii) the ATP-binding domain is not required for its activity as a holding chaperone, (iii) the β-sheet domain and the C-terminal α-helical cap appears to compose the substrate-binding pocket, (iv) the loop domain and the C-terminal cap are involved in the structural stability of the molecule. HSP110 proteins are important components of the eukaryotic HSP70 machinery of protein folding and act as nucleotide exchange factors and their mechanisms have been unveiled by Andreasson and collaborators. HSP110 protects heat-denatured proteins and confers cellular thermoresistance and is therefore identified as the principal chaperone of mammalian cells. Mammalian HSP110 also plays a significant role as RNA-binding entities *in vivo* to guide the appropriate folding substrates for subsequent regulatory processes of mRNA degradation or mRNA translation. The chaperoning properties of HSP110 have been exploited to construct a recombinant HSP110-HER-2/*neu* vaccine.

BiP/GRP78

Glucose-regulated protein 78 (GRP78) is one of the major chaperones localized mainly in the ER. Under normal physiological conditions, GRP78 is constitutively expressed as a resident protein of the ER and plays a significant role in protein folding in the ER lumen and protein translocation from the ER. The primary action of GRP78 is to ensure secretion of native proteins in their proper conformation by correctly folded tertiary and quaternary structures. GRP78 is an ATPase with a conserved ATPase domain and a peptide-binding domain. The ATPase catalytic site is located at the N-terminal domain and the ATPase activity is important for the *in vivo* function of GRP78. ATP hydrolysis induces a conformational change, enhancing the association of the C-terminal domain of GRP78 with its substrate. When ADP is exchanged for ATP again, the substrate is released and the chaperone cycle is completed. The weak ATPase activity is stimulated *in vitro* by small hydrophobic peptides that induce the release of GRP78 from bound polypeptides. Thereby, GRP78 is responsible for binding and release of the unfolded protein by repetitive hydrolysis of ATP hydrolysis and ADP exchange. Depletion of cellular ATP results in prolonged association with the protein. Short hydrophobic patches are exposed in incompletely folded proteins, misfolded proteins or unassembled subunits of oligomers and are selectively bound by GRP78 that exhibits its chaperoning activity. Functionally and structurally, it is similar to the HSP70 family including its binding affinity with ATP. However, they essentially diverge upon two distinct aspects: (i) GRP78 contains a signal peptide that targets it to the ER and (ii) it is not significantly induced upon other stress conditions that evoke the HSP response, but in particular to ER stress. GRP78 is also alternatively known as BiP, the immunoglobulin heavy chain-binding protein and it has been reported that it may also not be required for secretion of selective proteins. GRP78 is a significant ER stress protein that targets the Unfolded protein response (UPR) by mediating its effects on transmembrane proteins essential in UPR. Thus, it exerts UPR signaling and cell survival under ER stress. In normal conditions, GRP78 binds to three transmembrane proteins that act as transducers of ER stress signaling, PERK, IRE1 and ATF6 which are maintained in an inactive state. In their inactive forms, the N-termini of these transducers are held by GRP78 that prevents their aggregation. When misfolded proteins accumulate, GRP78 releases to allow aggregation of the proteins and thereby launching the UPR. Cell survival during ER stress is accomplished in UPR by inhibition of protein translation and activation of GRP78 expression that in turn inhibit apoptosis by interference with caspase activation. Of recent investigations, GRP78 is also known to be upregulated in early ischemic preconditioning and contributes towards cardioprotection.

ORP150/GRP170

Oxygen-regulated protein (ORP) of 150 kDa is analogous to the GRP170 glucose-regulated protein and is an ER chaperone of the HSP110 family. It is expressed constitutively in tissues with well-developed ER that are in active secretion of secretory proteins. This suggests its chaperoning functions in protein folding. ORP150 is specifically induced in hypoxia and enhances cellular ability to sustain oxygen deprivation. Bando and coworkers have suggested its ability to bind to ATP-agarose, a common structural affinity of HSPs. Recent investigations report their localization in mitochondria as well with cytoprotective and antiapoptotic activities and preservation of mitochondrial energy. ORP150 appears to play a plausible role in apoptosis, insulin secretion, protein transport and wound healing. The N-terminal half of ORP150 exhibits significant similarity with the ATPase domain of HSP70 family proteins with well-conserved ATP-binding motifs. The C-terminal is half-composed of a peptide-binding domain and an α-helical lid domain. Takeuchi has cloned the human heart ORP150 with a full-length 3301 bp sequence and a calculated MW of 111 kDa, with predicted 999 amino acid residues.

OSP94/ HSPA4L

OSP94 was first isolated in mouse renal medullary tissue with a putative amino-terminal ATP-binding domain and a putative carboxyl-terminal peptide-binding domain, showing 65% homology to HSP110 and 62% similarity with HSP70RY, thereby, belonging to the HSP110 family. An hypertonicity sensitive *cis*-acting element, OSP94-TonE was identified for expression of OSP94 upon osmotic stress that was distinct from a functional heat shock element (HSE). Recently, the authors have identified OSP94 as a biomarker of the human hypertensive heart tissue showing great homology and highly conserved sequence features among the mammalian stress proteins.

HSP70RY

HSP70RY belongs to the HSP110 subfamily and possesses structural features of molecular chaperones. This chaperone is expressed by an orphan gene in B-cells and shares homology to OSP94 with 62% identity.

2.1.2. HSP90

HSP90 is one of the most abundant constitutively expressed stress protein and is located in the nucleus and cytoplasm of eukaryotic cells. HSP90 is also heat-inducible and more strongly inducible by I/R injury. Generally, HSP90 is well-conserved among prokaryotes and in eukaryotes. HSP90 contains a catalytic loop that accepts the γ-phosphate of ATP in its core domain and is therefore characterized to be a split ATPase.

However, HSP90 is not capable of independent functionality as a protein chaperone, but requires the augmentation of its-co-chaperones. HSP90 is crucial in signal transduction to transformation to genetic capacitance and influences a wide array of cellular events. HSP90 comprises of three structural domains namely, an N-terminal domain that involves in ATP-binding, a proteolytically resistant core domain and a C-terminal domain that facilitates homodimerization.

A highly conserved pentapeptide MEEVD is present in the C-terminus of eukaryotic HSP90 which is recognized by its co-chaperones and therefore C-terminal domain also actively participates in the formation of functional HSP90 multiprotein complexes. In context of its structural architecture, HSP90 is a potent target for several promising lines of cancer therapeutics.

2.1.3. HSP70

HSP70 is the most abundant and best-characterized heat shock protein, first observed with hyperthermia. It has been observed that pre-induction of HSP70 by heat stress had various other beneficial effects after I/R injury. All members of the HSP70 family exhibit a common structure consisting of two domains; a highly conserved amino-terminal ATPase and a carboxy-terminal peptide-binding domain. HSP70 is also a powerful mediator of inflammation and immunity. However, conventional mechanisms do not aid HSP70 in traversing the plasma membrane, as it lacks a consensus secretory signal. Another mechanism of HSP70, independent of *de novo* synthesis or cell death is responsible for its active transport. HSP70 is effectively immunomodulatory in response to stress, and further, it also antagonizes the pro-inflammatory effects. More recently, HSP70 is shown to be a proven natural targeting system for APCs. Cytoplasmic delivery of HSP70–antigen further increased the efficacy of the HSP70-based vaccines. Henceforth, effective cancer therapy can be achieved by developing HSP70-based anticancer vaccines.

HSP72, an inducible form of the HSP70 family and is referred as a 'chaperokine' to describe its unique function as a chaperone as well as a cytokine. Intracellular HSP72 is generally cytoprotective by induction of the cells' anti-apoptotic mechanisms, repression of gene expression, modulation of cell cycle progression and anti-inflammation. Extracellular HSP72 is also immuno-stimulatory, stimulates pro-inflammatory cytokine synthesis, augments chemokine synthesis and enhances anti-tumor surveillance. HSP72 is released in a free form and within highly potent exosomes. HSP72 has a profound effect on host immunity and its circulation primes the immune system to real or perceived danger.

2.1.4. HSP60

HSP60 is constitutively expressed in the cytoplasm and translocated to the mitochondria. HSP60 is also heat inducible, although, ischemia has been shown to be a potent inducer. This class of stress proteins is a major molecular chaperone of the mitochondria. HSP60 facilitates the refolding of mitochondrial proteins as they translocate the inner and outer mitochondrial membranes. HSP60 consists of seven subunits with a weak K^+-dependent ATPase activity.

By constitutive expression, HSP60 also plays an essential role in normal cell function. In atherosclerotic models, autoimmunity to HSP60 indicated a plausible role in aetiology of the disease.

2.2. Small Heat Shock Proteins

The small HSP (sHSP) subfamily represent one of the best studied stress proteins and constitute a structurally divergent group characterized by a conserved sequence of 80-100 amino acid residues, with molecular masses ranging from 12-43 kDa and assemble into large dynamic complexes. In mammalian species, sHSPs comprise of: HSP27, HSPB1, HSPB2, HSPB3, αA-crystallin (HSPB4), αB-crystallin (HSPB5), HSP25, HSP20 (HSPB6), HSPB7, HSP22 (HSPB8), HSPB9 and HSPB10. The sHSPs have been classified into two main categories: Classes I and II, according to their different patterns of gene expression and subcellular localization.

All sHSPs share a common α-crystallin domain with unique N-terminal and C-terminal extensions and the latter is critical for their chaperone activity. sHSPs are molecular chaperones and act to prevent stress-induced protein aggregation of partially denatured proteins with restoration of their native conformational states. Perturbations of sHSP functions lead to cellular dysfunctions and eventual disease states due to metabolic turnover and protein degradation. Thereby, sHSPs maintain a normal cellular environment and perform vital metabolic functions that aid in a balanced hemostasis and cytoprotection.

HSP32, also a member of sHSP, plays a cytoprotective role and exerts antiinflammatory, antiapoptotic, antioxidant effects, and is also recently known to possess proangiogenic properties. HSP27 is involved in ATF5 (activating transcription factor 5)-mediated cell survival and increased cell tolerance. The α-crystallins share functional relevance with the sHSP family due to their high thermostability, phosphorylation patterns at specific Ser residues, tendency to form aggregates, exhibiting chaperone activity and protease inhibition, and association with cytoskeleton.

A novel small stress protein cvHSP of about 25 kDa abundantly expressed in human heart has been identified that shared an average of 26% and 49% identity and homology with six known sHSP members. Tissue distribution of cvHSP in human revealed that this stress protein is also expressed in skeletal muscle and adipose tissue.

2.3. Localization

The localization and functional activities of HSPs have a direct correlation in the context that subcellular location of HSPs affect the performance of their cellular functions in constitutive protein folding in the ER, inducible cytosolic protein refolding and prevention of protein aggregation and mitochondrial transportation of precursor proteins which have an influence on the overall metabolic and cellular activities.

Hence, depending on their localization in the cell, HSPs exhibit characteristic functions. Therefore, it is vital to observe their subcellular localization to derive at their predominant functional capabilities. We have presented the cellular location of HSP110 members and their functions in Table 2.1. Immunofluorescence and cell fractionation studies have revealed that HSP40 is mainly localized in the cytoplasm at normal growth temperatures and translocates into the nuclei and nucleoli upon heat shock and returns to cytoplasm.

Table 2.1. Localization of major HSP110 members

HSP class	Localization	Function
HSP110	Cytoplasm, Nucleus	Chaperone Nucleotide exchange factor Thermal resistance RNA binding
BiP/ GRP78	ER lumen ER transmembrane Cell surface Nucleus	Chaperone Ca^{2+} binding ER stress sensor UPR regulator Anti-apoptosis
ORP150/ GRP170	ER lumen Mitochondria	Chaperone Nucleotide exchange factor for GRP78 Hypoxia
OSP94/ HSPA4L	Cytoplasm Nucleus	Nucleotide binding ATP binding Protein folding Response to unfolded protein

It is also observed that HSP70 and HSP40 are colocalized and perform their functions in coherence. Members of HSP70 and HSP90 families have been frequently found to be located on the plasma membrane of a variety of tumor cells, while in normal tissues it is membrane negative. Thereby, HSPs have been found to play key roles in immunostimulation when located in the plasma membrane.

2.4. Gene Expression

Activation of the heat shockgene is rapid in response to heat stress or physiological stimuli. In the stressed cell, heat shock transcription factor (HSF) becomes phosphorylated and assembles to form activated trimers in the cytoplasm, accumulates in the nucleus, and associates with specific target sequences on the DNA promoter region of the heat-inducible gene, known as the heat shock element (HSE).

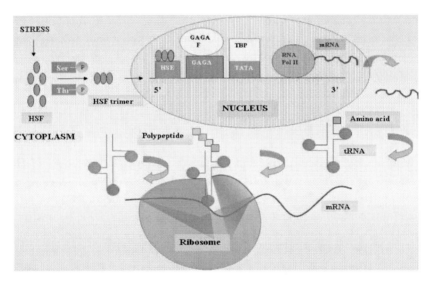

Figure 2.1. Mechanism of HSP gene expression. Upon stress, heat shock factors (HSF) accumulate in the cytoplasm and form active trimers by phosphorylation of Ser and Thr. HSF trimers traverse into the nucleus and bind to the heat shock element (HSE), a regulatory sequence upstream of the HSP gene, and activate RNA Pol II for synthesis of the mRNA transcript. The activation of RNA Pol II may also be effected by activation of GABA and TATA sequences by transcription factors GAGA factor (GAGAF) and TATA-binding protein (TBP). mRNA transcripts reach the cytoplasm where normal translation takes place in the ribosome unit with tRNAs.

The binding of the HSP trimer to the HSE results in transcription of HSP mRNA. Transcription of heat stress protein gene is also modulated by other transcription factors, such as, TATA-binding protein and the GAGA factor.

The next level of regulation occurs at translation of the heat shock protein mRNA. Heat shock genes do not contain introns or the intervening sequences, a unique feature of eukaryotic genes, which allow rapid transcription of the gene and mRNA processing. As a result, the response time for HSP expression is quick and efficient. Upon heat stress, HSP mRNA accumulatesin the cytoplasm, ribosomes bind to the template and HSPs are the products of protein synthesis.

2.5. Protein Folding

Endoplasmic reticulum (ER) is the major subcellular organelle distinctive of eukaryotic cells for protein secretion, while, it is periplasmic in case of prokaryotes. Following translation in the cytosol, proteins are translocated to the ER lumen, where glycosylation and folding occur and are subsequently released to the extracellular space where they perform their specific functions. Protein folding is assisted by a number of molecular chaperones and folding enzymes responsible for the maturation of nascent proteins in the ER lumen. We relate here some of the major chaperones in protein folding.

2.5.1. HSP70 and HSP40

While many classes of molecular chaperones co-exist, members of HSP70 and HSP40 are the most ubiquitous in folding of nascent polypeptides, prevention of protein denaturation and misfolding in cellular stress, degradation of proteins, protein translocation and quarternary assembly/disassembly. HSP70 consists of an N-terminal ATPase domain and a C-terminal substrate-binding domain. The affinity of HSP70 for precursor proteins is modulated by ATP binding and hydrolysis. HSP40 may bind the precursor proteins first and then target it to HSP70. HSP40 contains a 70 amino acid region known as the J-domain, essential for interaction with HSP70. The J-domain is a highly conserved α-helical structure that interacts with the HSP70 ATPase domain and possibly also with the HSP70 substrate-binding domain. Thereby, HSP70 and HSP40 cooperate as molecular chaperones to ensure fidelity at all stages of protein biogenesis.

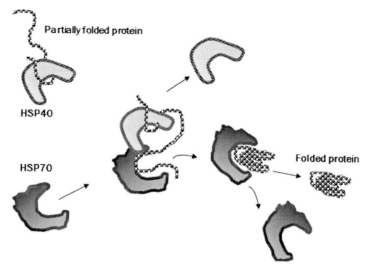

Figure 2.2. HSP70 and HSP40 in protein folding.

2.5.2. Calnexin (CNX) and Calreticulin (CRT)

CNX and CRT are well-characterized lectin chaperones of the mammalian ER which are homologous proteins with similar structure and function. CNX is membrane-anchored, while, CRT is present in the ER lumen. As nascent polypeptides enter the ER lumen, they are usually modified by N-glycans composed of two N-acetyl glucosamine, nine mannose and three glucose units. Glucosidases I and II immediately remove the glucose moieties. The terminal glucose residue of the oligosaccharide $[Glc_1Man_9GlcNAC_2]$ is critical for recognition by CNX/CRT. Removal of the last glucose destroys the binding site for these chaperones, thereby allowing the nascent protein to be transported to the Golgi if it has folded completely.

2.5.3. BiP/GRP78

GRP78/BiP is an ubiquitous resident protein of the ER lumen, which plays a key role in the assistance of newly synthesized proteins for protein folding and acquisition of correct tertiary and quarternary structure. BiP is an ATPase with its catalytic site located in the N-terminal domain. ATP hydrolysis induces a conformational change, which enhances the association of the C-terminal domain

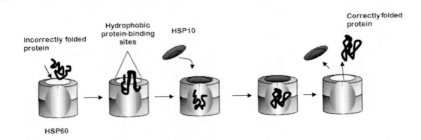

Figure 2.3. HSP60 and HSP10 in protein folding.

of BiP with its substrate. Upon phosphorylation of ADP into ATP, BiP releases its substrate and the chaperone cycle is completed. Activated BiP has several functions in protein translocation.

Initially, it is involved in the insertion of precursor polypeptides into the SEC61 complex of the protein translocase and opens up the channel by alteration of the conformation of the complex, where BiP interacts with GRP170. Secondly, BiP binds to the incoming precursor polypeptide and facilitates the completion of translocation. Finally, BiP is involved in the closure of the SEC61 channel, again, by alteration of the conformation of the complex.

2.5.4. HSP60

Arthur L.Horwich of YaleUniversityhas provided much of the current understanding of the HSP60 chaperone which resembles a cage composed of multiple HSP60 molecules.

Its inner rim is highly hydrophobic and therefore attracts the exposed hydrophobic amino acids of an unfolded protein to bind it. The polypeptide chain encounters a hydrophilic interior of the cage and being hydrophobic and repulsive, is forced to change shape and attain a native three-dimensional conformation and is released by the chaperone.

2.6. Apoptosis

Heat shock response is an intrinsic feature and tendency of most heat shock proteins to serve the stress overload by cellular adaptation in prevention of protein aggregation and inhibition of apoptosis and promote cell survival. Stress factors, environmental or physiological, evoke the protective responses of the heat shock proteins to aid in several mechanisms that contribute to the overall cellular functions.

Inhibition of apoptosis or the anti-apoptotic function is one of the major protective mechanisms offered by HSPs which act in a concerted fashion in a cascade of signaling pathways to inhibit the formation of the apoptosome. There also exist controversiesthat although heat shock proteins are molecular chaperones, their chaperoning functions are not essential for anti-apoptotic functions but by protein-protein interactions that are not yet well-understood.

The heat shock transcription factor, HSF1 is an important regulator of apoptosis. Any targeted disruption of this factor compromises with the apoptotic pathway and leads to cell death. A series of events that occur in apoptosis is given in Figure 2.4.

Inhibition of apoptosis by HSP induction occurs at the initiation site of mitochondrial release of cytochrome c. HSPs act at different stages in the apoptotic pathway thereby ensuring cellular protection by attacking many of its targets that contribute in the formation of the apoptosome.

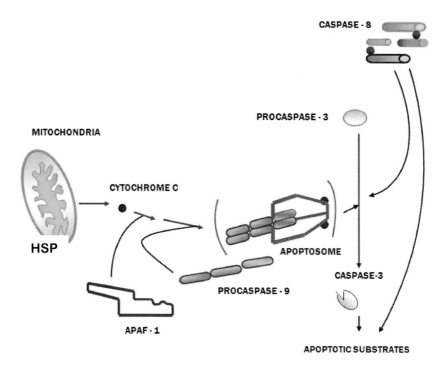

Figure 2.4. Apoptotic pathway.

Initially, HSPs block the effect of factors that induce cytochrome c secretion. Subsequent production of cytochrome c is again a substrate for inhibition by HSPs and another target is the binding of cytochrome c to Apaf1.

The next point of inhibition is Apaf1 by altering its structural conformation so as to prevent the binding of pro-caspase 9 to the Apaf1 complex. Thereby the formation of the apoptosome is completely inhibited.

HSP70-mediated inhibition of apoptosis has also been explained due to inhibition of activation of stress-activated protein kinase SAPK/JNK (c-Jun N-terminal kinase) signaling and its action downstream of caspase-3-like proteases. HSP70 or HSP90 act on Apaf1, while HSP27 inhibits the cytochrome c release.

Thereby, heat shock response to apoptosis is an efficient mechanism of cell survival and cytoprotection for maintenance of cellular hemostasis.

2.7. Codon Usage and GC Content Evolution

In a recent study, we have investigated the correlation of codon usage and GC content evolution of HSP110 members and have presented the results of such data to provide an understanding of the HSP110 ER members and cytosolic members in relation to BGC hypothesis.

2.7.1. Codon Usage

Codon usage has been correlated with the entire or partial nucleotide composition of the genome, gene expression levels and tissue-specific gene expression, as well as the degree of evolutionary amino acid conservation. Earlier studies show positive correlations between the nucleotide composition of genomic DNA and amino acid content of the encoded proteins.

Precisely, the codon first letter plays a dominant role in translating the genomic GC signature into protein amino acid composition and sequences while, there is a strong correlation between the GC content at third position of codons and the GC content of the region in which a gene is located.

This suggests that the distribution of GC content in mammals could have functional relevance. Furthermore, there is significant correlation between synonymous codon usage and protein secondary structure in the higher eukaryotes, particularly mammals.

2.7.2. Amino Acid Composition and GC Content

GC content of the member ORFs increase with an increase in GC3 in the mammalian HSP110 family (Figure 2.5).

This shows that preferred codons of the family ORFs usually end in C or G. In general, genes with a high codon usage bias tend to use a subset of the preferred codons rather than the full range of codons available. Previous studies have shown that increased GC content increases the amino acids (Pro, Ala, Arg, and Gly) encoded by GC-rich codons and decreases the amino acids (Phe, Ile, Met, Tyr, Asn, and Lys) encoded by GC-poor codons.

Concretely, residues of Pro, Ala, Arg, and Gly distributed a small range of approximately 4-9%, while residues of Phe, Ile, Met, Tyr, Asn, and Lys distributed a wide range of approximately 2-10% in the amino acid sequences of ER GRP78 and ORP150 (Figure 2.6).

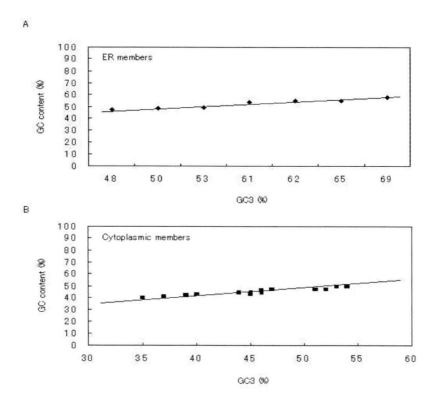

Figure 2.5. Correlation of GC3 with GC content of the mammalian HSP110 family. A, ER members B, Cytoplasmic members.

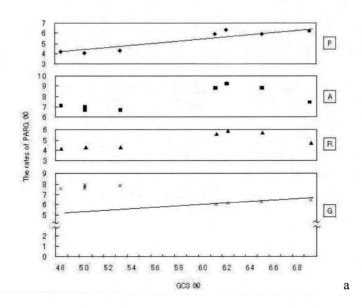

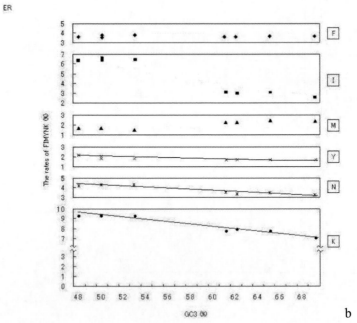

Firgure 2.6. (Continued).

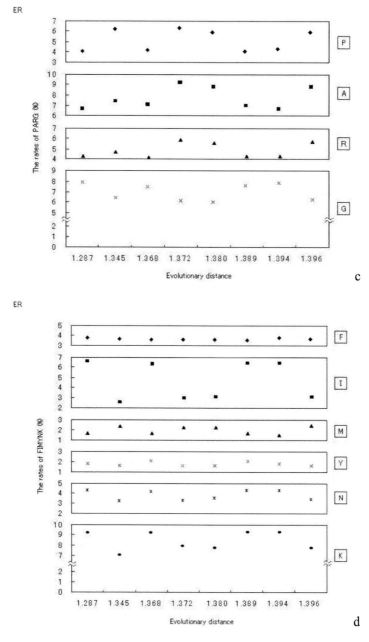

Figure 2.6. Correlation of rates of amino acids with GC3s and evolutionary distances of ER members. a, PARG rates vs. GC3s ; b, FIMYNK rates vs. GC3s ; c, PARG rates vs. evolutionary distance ; d, FIMYNK rates vs. evolutionary distance.

Figures 2.6.a. and 2.6.b. show correlations between the rates of amino acids (amino acid composition) encoded by GC-rich and GC-poor codons and the respective GC3s of the ER member ORFs. Residues of Pro and Gly increase with increasing GC3 (Figure 2.6.a) and the residues of Tyr, Asn, and Lys decrease with decreasing GC3 (Figure 2.6.b). Thus codon usage bias can be taken as a proxy for isochore composition. Thus, these results show that amino acid composition of the mammalian ER HSP110 family members have weak correlation with the GC3.

Figures 2.6.c. and 2.6.d. show correlations between the rates of amino acids encoded by GC-rich and GC-poor codons of the member ORFs and the evolutionary distance of the ER members. Evolutionary distance represents the branch point at which a given group diverges from all other groups and the most recently evolved groups are closest to the X-origin. These show that the amino acid composition has no correlation with the evolutionary distance in the ER members.

2.7.3. GC Content Evolution

GC content evolution in mammals follows the BGC hypothesis. Therefore, we investigated the correlation between the GC3s of GC-rich and GC-poor codons of the member ORFs and the evolutionary distance of the mammalian HSP110 family members. The results of ER members are depicted in Figure 2.7.

There was positive correlations, that, the GC3s of genetic codes for Pro and Ile residues increase with increasing evolutionary distance. On the other hand, the results of cytoplasmic members show no correlation between the GC3s of GC-rich and GC-poor codons of the member ORFs and the evolutionary distance of the members.

Thereby, mammalian ER HSP110 family members show a correlation of the ORFs of GRP78 and ORP150 between the amino acid composition encoded by GC-rich and GC-poor codons of the member ORFs and the GC3s while, there is lack of relevance with the mammalian cytoplasmic HSP110 family member ORFs. Interestingly, GC3s of genetic codes for hydrophobic amino acids (Val, Leu, Ile, and Pro) of ER members show positive correlation with the evolutionary distance of the ER members. These results suggest that the ER HSP110 family members in the mammalian HSP70 superfamily have independently evolved by increasing the GC3s of genetic codes for the Val, Leu, Ile, and Pro of hydrophobic amino acids that associate with protein stability, as well as the genomic influence of the ER members extends to the first and second codon positions. Consequently, our data support the BGC (biased gene conversion) hypothesis of GC content evolution also in the mammalian HSP110 family.

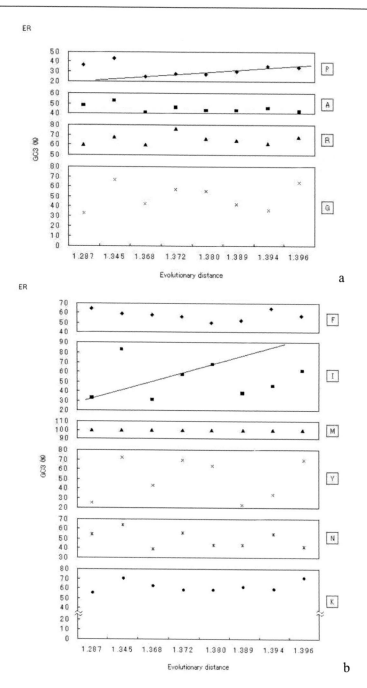

Figure 2.7. Correlation of GC3s with evolutionary distances of ER members. a, PARG GC3 vs. evolutionary distance ; b, FIMYNKGC3 vs. evolutionary distance.

References

Andreasson C, Fiaux J, Rampelt H, Druffel-Augustin S and Bukau B (2008) Insights into the structural dynamics of the HSP110-HSP70 interaction reveal the mechanism for nucleotide exchange activity. *PNAS* 105: 16519-16524.

Arrington DD and Schnellmann RG (2008) Targeting of the molecular chaperone oxygen-regulated protein 150 (ORP150) to mitochondria and its induction by cellular stress. *Am. J. Physiol. Cell Physiol.* 294: C641-C650.

Bando Y, Ogawa S, Yamauchi A, Kuwabara K, Ozawa K, Hori O, Yanagi H, Tamatani M, Tohyama M (2000) 150-kDa oxygen-regulated protein (ORP150) functions as a novel molecular chaperone in MDCK cells. *Am. J. Physiol. Cell Physiol.* 278: C1172-C1182.

Bernardi G (2000) Isochores and the evolutionary genomics of vertebrates. *Gene* 241: 3-17.

Calderwood SK, Theriault J, Gray PJ and Gong J (2007) Cell surface receptors for molecular chaperones. *Methods* 43: 199-206.

Dragovic Z, Broadley SA, Shomura Y, Bracher A and Hartl FU (2006) Molecular chaperones of the HSP110 family act as nucleotide exchange factors of HSP70s. *EMBO J.* 25: 2519-2528.

Flynn GC, Pohl J, Flocco MT and Rothman JE (1991) Peptide-binding specificity of the molecular chaperone BiP. *Nature* 353: 726-730.

Galtier N, Piganeau G, Mouchiroud D, Duret L (2001) GC-content evolution in mammalian genomes: The biased gene conversion hypothesis. *Genetics* 159: 907-911.

Gething MJ (1999) Role and regulation of the ER chaperone BiP. *Semin. Cell. Develop. Biol.*10: 465-472.

Hendershot LM (2004) The ER function BiP is a master regulator of ER function. *Mt.Sinai J. Med.* 71: 289-297.

Henics T, Nagy E, Oh HJ, Csermely P, von Gabain A and Subjeck JR (1999) Mammalian HSP70 and HSP110 proteins bind to RNA motifs involved in mRNA stability. *J. Biol. Chem.* 274: 17318-17324.

Hooper PL and Hooper JJ (2005) Loss of defence against stress: diabetes and heat shock proteins. *Diabetes Technol. Ther.*7: 204-208.

Hurst LD and Merchant AR (2001) High guanine-cytosine content is not an adaptation to high temperature: a comparative analysis amongst prokaryotes. *Proc. Biol. Sci.* 268: 493–497.

Ikeda J, Kaneda S, Kuwabara K, Ogawa S, Kobayashi T, Matsumoto M, Yura T and Yanagi H (1997) Cloning and expression of cDNA encoding the human150 kDa oxygen-regulated protein, ORP150. *Biochem. Biophys. Res. Commun.* 230: 94–99.

Iwaki A, Nagano T, Nakagawa M, Iwaki T and Fukumaki Y (1997) Identification and characterization of the gene encoding a new member of the α-crystallin/small hsp family, closely linked to the αB-crystallin gene in a head-head manner. *Genomics* 45: 386-394.

Kleizen B and Braakman I (2004) Protein folding and quality control in the endoplasmic reticulum. *Curr. Opinion Cell Biol.* 16: 343-349.

Kobayashi T and Ohta Y (2005) 150-kDa oxygen-regulated protein is an essential factor for insulin release. *Pancreas* 30: 299-306.

Kojima R, Randall J, Brenner BM and Gullans SR (1996) Osmotic stress protein 94 (OSP94)-A new member of the HSP110/SSE gene subfamily. *J. Biol. Chem.* 271: 12327-12332.

Kojima R, Randall JD, Ito E, Manshio H, Suzuki Y and Gullans SR (2004) Regulation of expression of the stress response gene, OSP94: Identification of the tonicity response element and intracellular signaling pathways. *Biochem. J.* 380: 783-794.

Kreif S, Faivrei JF, Robert P, Douarin BL, Brument-Larignon N, Lefrere I, Bouzyk MM, Anderson KM, Greller LD, Tobin FL, Souchet M and Bril A (1999) Identification and characterization of cvHSP.A novel human small stress protein selectively expressed in cardiovascular and insulin-sensitive tissues. *J. Biol. Chem.* 274: 36592-36600.

Kumarapeli ARK and Wang X (2004) Genetic modification of the heart: chaperones and the cytoskeleton. *J. Mol. Cell. Cardiol.* 37:1097-1109.

Kuwabara K, Matsumoto M, Ikeda J, Hori O, Ogawa S, Maeda Y, Kitagawa K, Imuta N, Kinoshita T, Stern DM, Yanagi H and Kamada T (1996) Purification and characterization of a novel stress protein, the 150-kDa oxygen-regulated protein (ORP150), from cultured rat astrocytes and its expression in ischemic mouse brain*J. Biol.Chem.* 271: 5025-5032.

Lee AS (2005) The ER chaperone and signaling regulator GRP78/BiP as a monitor of endoplasmic reticulum stress. *Methods* 35: 373-381.

Lee-Yoon D, Easton D, Murawski M, Burd R and Subjeck JR (1995) Identification of a major subfamily of large hsp70-like proteins through the cloning of the mammalian 110-kDa heat shock protein. *J. Biol.Chem.*270: 15725-15733.

Levinson W, Oppermann H and Jackson J (1980) Transition series metals and sulfhydryl reagents induce the synthesis of four proteins in eukaryotic cells. *Biochim. Biophys. Acta* 606: 170-180.

Mala JGS and Takeuchi S (2008) Heat shock proteins in cardiovascular stress. *Clin.Med:Cardiol* 2: 245-256.

Mala JGS and Takeuchi S (2008) Molecular chaperones of mammalian ER in protein folding and quality control. In: *Heat shock proteins: New Research*, ed. Morel E and Vincent C, Nova Publishers, USA, pp.1-27.

Mala JGS and Takeuchi S (2009) Molecular cloning of OSP94: A significant biomarker protein of hypertensive human heart and a member of HSP110 family. *Mol. Biotechnol.* 42: 175-194.

Manjili MH, Henderson R, Wang X-Y, Chen X, Li Y, Repasky E, Kazim L and Subjeck JR (2002) Development of a recombinant HSP110-HER-2/*neu* vaccine using the chaperoning properties of HSP110. *Cancer Res.* 62: 1737-1742.

Morris JA, Dorner AJ, Edwards CA, Hendershot LM and Kaufman RJ (1997) Immunoglobulin binding protein (BiP) function is required to protect cells from endoplasmic reticulum stress but is not required for the secretion of selective proteins. *J. Biol. Chem.* 272: 4327-4334.

Multhoff G (2007) Heat shock protein 70 (HSP70): Membrane location, export and immunological relevance. *Methods* 43: 229-237.

Munro S and Pelham HRB (1986) An hsp70-like protein in the ER: Identity with the 78 kd glucose-regulated protein and immunoglobulin heavy chain binding protein. *Cell* 46: 291-300.

Ni M and Lee AS (2007) ER chaperones in mammalian development and human diseases. *FEBS Lett*581: 3641-3651.

Oh HJ, Chen X and Subjeck JR (1997) HSP110 protects heat denatured proteins and confers cellular thermoresistance. *J. Biol. Chem.* 272: 31636-31640.

Oh HJ, Easton D, Murawski M, Kaneko Y and Subjeck JR (1999) The chaperoning activity of HSP110-Identification of functional domains by use of targeted deletions.*J. Biol. Chem.* 274: 15712-15718.

Ohtsuka K and Hata M (2000) Molecular chaperone function of mammalian HSP70 and HSP40-a review. *Int.J.Hyperthermia* 16: 231-245.

Ozawa K, Kondo T, Hori O, Kitao Y, Stern DM (2001) Eisenmenger, W., Ogawa, S. and Ohshima, T. Expression of the oxygen-regulated protein ORP150 accelerates wound healing by modulating intracellular VEGF transport. *J. Clin. Invest.* 108: 41-50.

Ozawa K, Kuwabara K, Tamatani M, Takatsuji K, Tsukamoto Y, Kaneda S, Yanagi H, Stern DM, Eguchi Y, Tsujimoto Y, Ogawa S and Tohyama M (1999) 150-kDa oxygen-regulated protein (ORP150) suppresses hypoxia-induced apoptotic cell death. *J. Biol. Chem.* 274: 6397-6404.

Pockley AG, Fairburn B, Mirza S, Slack LK, Hopkinson K and Muthana M (2007) A non-receptor-mediated mechanism for internalization of molecular chaperones. *Methods* 43: 238-244.

Porter TD (1995) Correlation between codon usage, regional genomic nucleotide composition, and amino acid composition in the cytochrome P-450 gene superfamily. *Biochim. Biophys. Acta* 1261: 394–400.

Riezman H (2004) Why do cells require heat shock proteins to survive heat stress? *Cell Cyc.* 3: 61-63.

Shintani-Ishida K, Nakajima M, Uemura K and Yoshida K (2006) Ischemic preconditioning protects cardiomyocytes against ischemic injury by inducing GRP78. *Biochem. Biophys. Res. Commun.* 345: 1600-1605.

Singer GA and Hickey DA (2000) Nucleotide bias causes a genomewide bias in the amino acid composition of proteins. *Mol. Biol. Evol.* 17: 1581–1588.

Srivastava PK (2008) New jobs for ancient chaperones. *Sci.Am.India*, July, pp.36-41.

Sun Y and MacRae TH (2005) The small heat shock proteins and their role in human disease. *FEBS J.* 272: 2613-2627.

Takeuchi S (2006) Molecular cloning, sequence, function and structural basis of human heart 150 kDa oxygen-regulated protein, an ER chaperone. *The Protein J.* 25: 517-528.

Tao Xand Dafu D (1998) The relationship between synonymous codon usage and protein structure. *FEBS Lett.* 434: 93-96.

van Anken E and Braakman I (2005) Versatility of the endoplasmic reticulum protein folding factory. *Crit. Rev. Biochem. Mol. Biol.* 40: 191-228.

Wang H, Lin G and Zhang Z (2007) ATF5 promotes cell survival through transcriptional activation of HSP27 in H9c2 cells. *Cell Biol. Int.* 31: 1309-1315.

Wilquet V and de Casteele MV (1999) The role of the codon first letter in the relationship between genomic GC content and protein amino acid composition. *Res. Microbiol.* 150: 21-32.

Wolfe KH, Sharp PMand Li WH (1989) Mutation rates differ among regions of the mammalian genome. *Nature* 337: 283–285.

Xu C, Bailly-Maitre B and Reed JC (2005) Endoplasmic reticulum stress: cell life and death decisions. *J. Clin. Invest.* 115: 2656-2664.

In: Heat Shock Proteins …   ISBN: 978-1-61324-589-7
Authors: S. Takeuchi and J. G. S. Mala   © 2012 Nova Science Publishers, Inc.

Chapter III

Cardiovascular Diseases

Abstract

Mankind is highly associated with cardiovascular diseases since centuries past. In today's world, there has been a constant awareness on heart ailments and research based diagnostics have shown to have decreased the mortality rate and an average man's life span has been extended to 60-70 years. Rejuvenative and preventive measures are on the rise in today's stride towards a healthy heart. Inspite of the renaissance, poor lifestyle values and sedentary mode of living have also led to a rapid increase of an average individual to be susceptible to cardiovascular disorders. Fatty foods and unhealthy food habits have contributed to a marked rise in heart problems as predicted by WHO for about 10-15 years ahead. A precise knowledge of the diseases of the heart is therefore described as a prelude to the different heat shock protein responses in cardiovascular stress discussed in Chapter 4.

3.1. The Cardiovascular System

The cardiovascular system is the fundamental and important organ in the human system and plays a major role in normal functioning of the entire human body. A perturbation of this system leads to cardiovascular disorders which can be fatal and hence require investigations of the maintenance of its primary functions and normal rhythm. The heart and the associated blood vessels with proper functioning of the circulation system are a concerted approach for speculation by researchers worldwide. Cardiovascular disease (CVD) is a debilitating illness arising from genetic predisposition and socio-economic relevance. Decades earlier, CVD were common in the Western population, but have evolved in recent years to the Asian race, and therefore depend on ethnic background. The quality of life or the routine lifestyle of an individual is a fundamental factor in developing heart ailments. Since the millennium, there has been a surge of awareness among the modern population by the media which also prescribe a healthy diet to overcome dietary risk factors. A major concern is age-related risk factors that show little or no effect to undertake preventive measures and it is essential that heart consciousness starts right above 35 years of age for both men and women. Hence, we have dedicated this chapter to the significance of the heart structure and function and its susceptibility to various stress factors resulting in CVD. Major heart abnormalities are elicited here which evoke significant HSP response.

3.1.1. Heart

The heart is a muscular organ in size of about the clenched fist of the individual. It is located in the inner chest of the upper part of the body with its apex pointing towards the left.

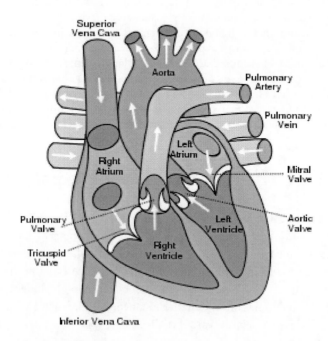

Figure 3.1. C.S of human heart.

The primary function of the heart is to pump blood backwards and forwards within the heart receiving and discharging blood and never stops until death, every minute, and every fraction of seconds. The cross section of the human heart structure is depicted in Figure 3.1.

The heart is enclosed in a double-layered fibrous sheath, the pericardium which prevents enlargement of the heart muscle. The outer layer of the heart, the epicardium is a layer of mesothelial cells while the inner layer endocardium consists of endothelial cells similar to blood vessels.

The heart muscle is the myocardium which aids in the rigorous pumping of blood. The interstitial space in between the epicardium and the pericardium is the pericardial fluid that serves as a lubricant to avoid frictions of the heart muscle. The heart consists of four chambers divided into the right and left atrium and the right and left ventricles.

The right atrium receives impure blood (about 70% saturation) from the superior and inferior vena cava from the systemic circulation and is passed on to the right ventricle via the tricuspid valve. The right ventricle forwards the impure (deoxygenated) blood to the pulmonary arteries via the pulmonary semilunar valves which takes the blood to the lungs for purification of blood known as oxygenation.

The oxygenated blood with about 98% saturation reaches the left atrium through pulmonary veins. A notable paradox is the classification of the passage of deoxygenated blood in pulmonary artery and the return of the oxygenated blood in the pulmonary veins since arteries generally transport pure blood and veins transport impure blood.

Ventricular filling occurs through the mitral valve (bicuspid) which is then pumped out into the aorta, the major artery in the circularory system via the aortic semilunar valve which closes when the ventricular pressure falls to prevent backflow of the blood from the aorta into the left ventricle.

Relaxation of the heart occurs for filling of blood while heart muscle contracts to pump out the blood. The aorta supplies blood (oxygenated) to all the tissues from the head to trunk and pelvis to legs, through smaller arteries, arterioles and the capillaries. The coronary artery supplies blood to the heart.

It can be observed that the left ventricular muscle is twice or thrice thicker than any of the other chambers as it has to work harder to pump the blood to the entire system. In an average life span, the heart pumps about 1 million barrels of blood. During stress or exercise, the heart pumps as much as 10 times than at rest.

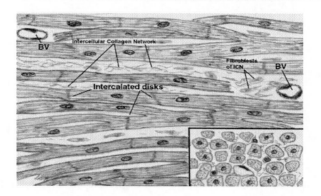

Figure 3.2. Histology of myocardium (C.S. in Inset).

3.1.2. Myocardium

The myocardium is an involuntary striated muscle made up of cardiac cells known as cardiomyocytes which appear in structure and function intermediate to the skeletal muscle and the smooth muscle cells (Figure 3.2). The cells are relatively small of about $100x20\mu m$ and branched, with a single nucleus and rich in mitochondria, connected to each other by intercalated discs where the cell membranes are closely opposed. The presence of abundant mitochondria helps in the energy requirements of the myocardial muscle. The intercalated discs provide both structural attachment and an electrical connection and hence the myocardium functions as a single entity. The cardiomyocytes are composed of actin and myosin filaments and the myocardium has an extensive system of capillaries.

3.1.3. Cardiac Cycle

The sequence of the mechanical events in a single heart beat is termed the cardiac cycle by which electrical activity coordinates with rhythmic relaxation and contraction of the atria and the ventricles. These two phases are distinguished as diastole when the ventricles relax and the systole when the ventricles undergo contraction. During diastole, the two atria contract driven by an impulse from the sinus node and the tricuspid and mitral valves open and fills up the relaxed ventricles. The end of diastole triggers the contraction of the ventricles by the electrical impulse.Systole of the ventricles closes the tricuspid and mitral valves and blood is ejected from the right ventricle into the pulmonary artery and from the left ventricle into the aorta.

The subsequent relaxation of the ventricles pushes down the blood from pulmonary artery and aorta which close down the pulmonary valve and the aortic valve to prevent backflow of the blood. Ventricular pressure is then lower than in the atria which open up the tricuspid and mitral valves and forces blood from the two atria into the relaxed ventricles and the cycle continues. The entire cycle takes about approximately one second. Diastole is the longer phase which takes two-thirds of the cardiac cycle while systole takes about one-third.

3.1.4. Blood Pressure

Blood flow traverses the entire circulatory system through blood vessels such as arteries and aterioles. The flow of blood exerts force on the surface of the artery walls to keep it moving along the blood vessels and is referred as blood pressure. The pressure arises from the heart but it is greatly felt in the arteries and smaller arterioles which actually determine the amount of pressure. The blood vessels constrict to raise the blood pressure (vasoconstriction) and dilate to lower the blood pressure (vasodilation). There are a many number of effectors that cause vasoconstriction and vasodilation to aid in regulation of the blood pressure. In an individual, the arterial pressure is determined by the cardiac output and the total peripheral resistance (TPR), which vary widely among individuals and within one individual at different times. The normal blood pressure of a resting individual is 120/80 mm Hg. The blood pressure averages about 80/60 mmHg at birth and rises slowly throughout childhood. In an adolescent, the resting blood pressure is in the order of 120/70 mmHg, while in the middle age, 140/80 mmHg is common. The mean pressure during sleep may be 30 mm Hg lower than the normal pressure. At exercise, the systolic pressure rises up considerably with little or no effect in diastole. Thus, marked variations in blood pressure occur in different physical activities of an individual and factors such as anxiety and emotional stress also add to the pressure load.

3.2. Cardiovascular Risk Factors

Cardiovascular risk factors are markers, the presence or levels of which correlate with future probabilities of cardiovascular diseases (CVD) and/death in an individual.

Table 3.1. Cardiovascular risk factors

Fixed factors	Modifiable factors
Age	High cholesterol, Low HDL
	Hypertension, Chronic kidney disease
Gender	Diabetes mellitus
Genetic predisposition	Dyslipidaemia (LDL, lipoprotein a)
	Vitamin D deficiency
	Salt sensitivity
	Left ventricular hypertrophy
	Obesity
	Tobacco smoking, excessive alcohol
	Sedentary lifestyle
	Drug abuse (cocaine, methamphetamine)

A list of risk factors has been proposed by the Framingham Heart study from 1948-1970 in Framingham, Massachusetts, USA that predispose the individual to the likelihood of acquiring CVD. Table 3.1 lists many of the risk factors from the Framingham heart study to the present research findings. Depending on gender and heredity and physiological and metabolic factors, the cardiovascular risk factors are grouped as fixed or modifiable factors. Protective factors that promote cardioprotection are HDL (high density lipoprotein) cholesterol, exercise, estrogen and moderate alcohol intake.

3.3. Cardiovascular Diseases

Cardiovascular disease is a leading health problem in the Western world.A marked increase in the cardiovascular risk factors lead to atherosclerosis, plaque rupture, thrombosis, myocardial infarction and heart failure by interdependent clinical modulations (Figure 3.3).

3.3.1. Myocardial Infarction

Myocardial infarction (MI) is necrosis of heart tissue caused by ischemia or an atherosclerotic plaque rupture in the coronary artery. Acute myocardial infarction (AMI) arises when a localized myocardial ischemia causes necrotic cell death (Fig.3.4). MI is most commonly due to occlusionof a coronary arteryfollowing the rupture of a vulnerable atherosclerotic plaque, which is an unstable collection of lipids and white blood cells (macrophages) in the wall of an artery. The resulting ischemia and oxygen shortage, if left untreated for a sufficient period of time, can cause damage or death (infarction) of the myocardium. The mortality and morbidity of MI is significantly a consequence of the infarct size and the coronary occlusion formed by thrombus, an internal clot that plugs the coronary artery.

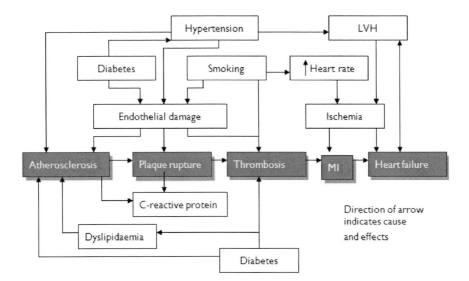

Figure 3.3. Interactions of risk factors leading to CVD.

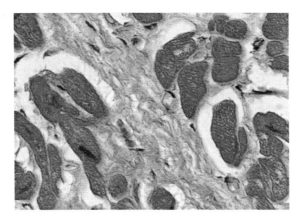

Figure 3.4. Myocardial infarction showing necrotic tissue.

There are two basic types of acute myocardial infarction, (1) transmural MI-associated with atherosclerosis involving major coronary artery, (2) subendocardial MI- localised in the subendocardial wall of the left ventricle, ventricular septum, papillary muscles. Clinically, based on ECG changes, myocardial infarction is further subclassified into ST elevation MI and non-ST elevation MI.

Pathophysiology of MI

Ischemia is loss or restricted blood supply which progresses as an infarct leading to necrosis of part or whole of the myocardium. The clinical development of an infarct thus starts from ischemic loss of contractility in the affected myocardium. Necrosis starts to develop in 15-20 min after coronary occlusion in the subendocardium which is more prone to ischemia and extends towards the epicardium in 3-6 h and eventually spans the entire ventricular wall. Cellular, histological and gross changes occur within the infarct showing abnormalities in cell biochemistry and ultrastructure. Progressive cell damage becomes increasingly irreversible over 12 h, providing a survival time span for thrombolysis and reperfusion to salvage some of the infarct. Coagulation necrosis characterized by cell swelling, organelle breakdown and protein denaturation in the infarcted myocardium is followed by a rapid neutrophil infiltration in about 18 h. Granulation tissue appears at the infarct edges consisting of macrophages and fibroblasts that lay down a scar tissue and new capillaries and in a period of 2-3 months, the infarct leaves a thinned, firm and pale grey noncontracting region of the ventricular wall. Infarct expansion leads to ventricular remodeling which is subject to cardiovascular risk with subsequent development of congestive heart failure and ventricular arrhythmia.

Coronary thrombosis (Fig.3.5) from an atherosclerotic lesion is a critical event leading to MI. Coronary plaques contain a large lipid-rich core covered by a thin fibrous cap.

Activated macrophages and T-lymphocytes release metalloproteases and cytokines to weaken the fibrous cap rendering it liable to rupture due to the shear stress exerted by the bloodflow. Plaque rupture reveals subendothelial collagen, a site for platelet adhesion, activation and aggregation. The degree of coronary occlusion and myocardial damage caused by plaque rupture depends on systemic catecholamine levels, plaque location and morphology, depth of plaque rupture and extent of coronary vasoconstriction.

Severe and prolonged ischemia causes a transmural infarct that produces ST segment elevation, while, less severe and protracted ischemia limits the infarct to the subendocardium and produces a typical non-ST segment elevation MI.

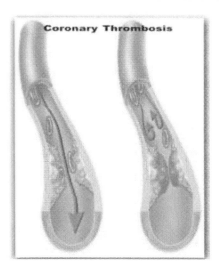

Figure 3.5. Coronary artery forming thrombosis.

3.3.2. Heart Failure

Heart failure is one of the leading causes of death occurring in 2-3% of the general population and with >10% prevalence in older patients above 65 years. Clinically, heart failure is the condition of the heart when it stops pumping blood due to an inadequate cardiac output and cardiac function eventually declines. Thereby, the structure or function of the heart impairs its ability to supply sufficient blood flow to meet the body's needs. Common causes of heart failure include myocardial infarction and other forms of ischemic heart disease, hypertension, valvular heart disease and cardiomyopathy. Heart failure may be acute with a rapid onset and decompensated heart while chronic condition lasts for a longer period. Systolic failure is a defect in heart function that imapirs ejection of flow of blood. Diastolic failure is a defect in ventricular filling causing a preload, that is an elevated filling pressure. Heart failure also occurs when the heart muscle is disordered. The American Heart Association in its 2001 guidelines has introduced four stages that a patient would succumb to heart failure:

Stage A: Patients at high risk for developing HF in the future but no functional or structural heart disorder

Stage B: a structural heart disorder but no symptoms at any stage

Stage C: previous or current symptoms of heart failure in the context of an underlying structural heart problem, but managed with medical treatment

Stage D: advanced disease requiring hospital-based support, a heart transplant or palliative care

New York Heart Association Functional Classification of heart failure are:

Class I: no limitation is experienced in any activities; there are no symptoms from ordinary activities

Class II: slight, mild limitation of activity; the patient is comfortable at rest or with mild exertion

Class III: marked limitation of any activity; the patient is comfortable only at rest

Class IV: any physical activity brings on discomfort and symptoms occur at rest

Pathophysiology of Heart Failure

The modulations and responses in pathophysiology of heart failure is depicted in Figure 3.6. Left heart failure occurs as a consequence of a prior ischemic heart disease.

Decreased cardiac output leads to preload and an increase in pulmonary venous pressure causing the heart to dilate and promote fluid accumulation in the lung interstitiumdue to increased pulmonary capillary pressure causing dyspnoea or breathlessness. A severe rise in the capillary pressure retreats fluid collection in the alveoli causing pulmonary edema, highly, a life threatening condition.

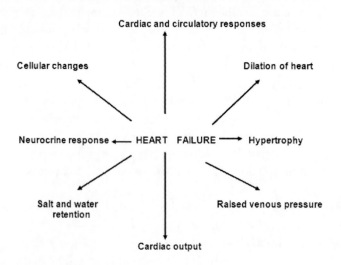

Figure 3.6. Implications of Heart Failure.

The increased pulmonary vascular pressure leads to pressure overload and failure of the right heart, a case of congestive heart failure. Right heart failure alone can be caused by chronic lung disease, pulmonary hypertension or embolism and valve disease.

3.3.3. Hypertension

Hypertension is a cardiovascular disorder with an increase in blood pressure of a resting individual, usually higher than 150/90 mm Hg. Hypertension is a major risk factor for CVD, leading to stroke, infarction, renal failure and congestive heart failure. Essential or Primary hypertension is a multifactorial genetic disorder, in which an inheritance of a number of abnormal genes predisposes an individual to high blood pressure, when appropriate stimuli are also present. Identification of the causative genes presently remains unresolved but has led to observations of functional abnormalities associated with hypertension. Thereby, the specific causes are not defined; however, it may relate to genetic predisposition, dietary factors such as high salt intake, physical stress, hormonal disturbances and increased cardiac output. Vascular smooth muscle cell proliferation and hypertrophy are the hall marks of hypertension. Oxidative stress is a significant factor affecting hypertension and is also associated with vascular damage. Hypertension is therefore a progressive disease leading to cell death and eventually heart failure. Hypertension is attributed to a known cause or disorder in <10% cases and is classified as Secondary hypertension which result from renovascular disease, endocrine malfunctions and use of oral contraceptives. Accelerated hypertension is an uncommon malignant form of the disease which rapidly affects the retina, kidneys, brain and heart and causes premature death.

Pathophysiology of Hypertension

Hypertension arises from peripheral vascular resistance with alterations in structure, mechanical properties and function of small arteries. The vasculature is an integral organ affected by hypertension. In early stages of essential hypertension, the cardiac output and viscosity of blood are normal with an increase in arteriolar muscle tone with subsequent structural alterations in the arterioles. Therefore, a removal of the cause of hypertension does not necessarily lead to normal blood pressure. Sustained hypertension leads to two major consequences in the heart, heart failure and atherosclerosis. An increased function of the hypertensive heart results in hypertrophy of the myocardial cells. This progresses to a disruption of coronary blood supply in the subendocardial layers of the heart muscle and deposition of fibrous tissue leading to reduced ventricular compliance and ultimately heart failure. Atherosclerosis occurs in coronary arteries, cerebral arteries and renal arteries although the mechanisms are unclear. Racial discrimination of hypertension has been observed with black patients contracting severe left ventricular hypertrophy, while whites generally show consequences of atherosclerosis. Cardiac cells of hypertensive patients result in accelerated metabolic rate leading to increased ageing.A study of clinical importance in women has indicated that ischemic disease and stroke increase progressively and linearly with increasing degree of hypertension. The pathogenesis of hypertension relates to the renin-angiotensin system (RAS) which modulate pressure-natriuresis in normal physiology and in disease states (Fig. 3.7). Hypertensive tissues, heart and kidney respond to the osmotic imbalance caused by an impairment of the RAS leading to increased sodium reabsorption which influences the body fluid volume, a critical factor affecting the intra arterial pressure. Thereby sodium reabsorption and consequent osmotic imbalance have a direct role on the cause and effect of hypertension.

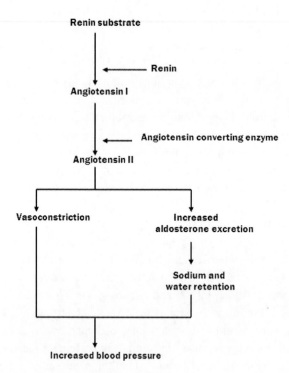

Figure 3.7. Renin-Angiotensin System.

3.3.4. Cardiomyopathy

Cardiomyopathy is a disease of the heart muscle. Primary cardiomyopathy is a disease confined to the heart not arising from an identifiable disease process, while Secondary cardiomyopathy is a disease of the heart muscle due to a generalized systemic disorder. Commonly, heart muscle disease is a result of damage caused by myocardial infarction, and maybe referred as Ischemic cardiomyopathy, however, varying in the focal nature of myocardial abnormality. Cardiomyopathy may be classified depending upon the functional impairment observed: dilated, hypertrophic or restrictive. Dilated cardiomyopathy is not a single disease entity, but is an end result of myocardial damage caused by different mechanisms and is familial and family history should be taken into consideration during diagnosis. Hypertrophic cardiomyopathy is a massive hypertrophy of the ventricles with an increased stiffness of the left ventricle resulting in impaired diastolic filling leading to pulmonary congestion. Dyspnoea is a common symptom of this disease. Restrictive cardiomyopathy is an abnormal stiffening of the ventricles and impedes ventricular filling leading to impaired diastolic function. Systolic function may remain normal.

Pathophysiology of Cardiomyopathy

Dilated ventricles increase the pressure in left atrium with subsequent occurrence of pulmonary hypertension and right ventricular failure in dilated cardiomyopathy. Impaired diastolic function is a common abnormality and minimally symptomatic or asymptomatic clinical features may be identified in hypertrophic cardiomyopathy. Infiltration of the myocardium or endomyocardial scarring is a secondary pathological feature of restrictive cardiomyopathy.

References

Aaronson PI, Ward JPT and Wiener CM (2005) The Cardiovascular system at a glance (2nd ed.), Blackwell Publishing, USA.

Dzau VJ, Gibbons GH, Morishita R, and Pratt RE (1994) New perspectives in hypertension research. Potentials of vascular biology. *Hypertension*23: 1132-1140.

Hall, JE, Granger JP, Reckelhoff JF and Sandberg K (2008) Hypertension and cardiovascular disease in women. *Hypertension*51: 951.

Julian DG, Cowan JC and McLenachan JM (2007) *Cardiology*, (5th ed.), Saunders Elsevier, USA.

Oparil S, Zaman MA and Calhoun DA (2003) Pathogenesis of hypertension. *Ann. Intern. Med.*139: 761-776.

Touyz RM (2004) Reactive oxygen species, vascular oxidative stress and redox signaling in hypertension: What is the clinical significance? *Hypertension*44: 248-252.

Ushio-Fukai M, Alexander RW, Akers M and Griendling KK (1998) p38 mitogen-activated protein kinase is a critical component of the redox-sensitive signaling pathways activated by angiotensin II-role in vascular smooth muscle cell hypertrophy. *J. Biol. Chem.*273: 15022-15029.

Zheng Y, Im CN and Seo JS (2006) Inhibitory effect of HSP70 on angiotensin II-induced vascular smooth muscle cell hypertrophy. *Exptl. Mol. Med.*38: 505-518.

In: Heat Shock Proteins …   ISBN: 978-1-61324-589-7
Authors: S. Takeuchi and J. G. S. Mala   © 2012 Nova Science Publishers, Inc.

Chapter IV

Heat Shock Proteins in Cardioprotection

Abstract

The human heart has been associated with heat shock protein expression since Murry and his coworkers described the effects of ischemic preconditioning in 1986. Heat shock protein response in cardiovascular ailments is a prerequisite for cardioprotection and the many number of HSPs contribute towards targeting cellular mechanisms for cell survival and preclude the cardiac stress. In this Chapter, we focus on the various cardioprotective effects of HSPs in a number of cardiac clinical presentations, their potential mechanisms and cellular responses. We have also provided a vivid account of the regulation of HSP expression by signaling pathways which mediate cardioprotection from pertinent literature available.

4.1. Heat Shock Proteins and Heart

The heart is the primary target of cardiovascular illness and responds to stress by an upregulation of heat shock proteins, chaperones that act to mediate cardioprotection. The rapid induction of HSPs is crucial for cell survival and is a central conserved feature in bacteria to humans. The primary function of HSPs in stressed and normal conditions is to assist polypeptide chain folding and assembly into tertiary and quartenary structures to form native conformational states. Protein unfolding and aggregation elicit a powerful transient accumulation of

HSPs that promote cytoprotection. HSPs either prevent protein aggregation of unfolded proteins or solubilize existing aggregates. If the cytosolic protein folding exceeds the threshold or the basal capacity of chaperone networks by environmental or metabolic stress factors, the 'unfolded protein response' comes into effect in the ER. Denatured and misfolded proteins that are unable to be repaired by the chaperones are efficiently targeted for removal by intracellular proteolysis known as the 'ubiquitin-proteasome machinery'. Thereby, HSPs act in a concerted fashion first in stabilizing protein folding, aid in refolding of unfolded proteins, prevent protein aggregation by sensing and responding to cellular stress.

CVD is a manifestation of cardiac stress arising from physiological, environmental and pathological stress stimuli. The cause and effects of stress stimuli are classified as the risk factors for CVD. Cardiovascular risk factors have been evaluated in Chapter III (Table 3.1 and Fig.3.3). It has been recently discussed that high normal blood pressure and anti-HSP27 antibody levels are also grouped as cardiovascular risk factors. In 2007, the guidelines for management of hypertension considered the division of high-normal blood pressure subjects as in prehypertension status which might progress into hypertension over time. Along with the West, Japan is in the line of higher cases of CVDs and in 2009, the Japanese guidelines has considered diabetes, chronic kidney disease, 3 or more risk factors and target organ damage as a high-risk group even with high-normal blood pressure and has prescribed antihypertensive therapy. In 2008, Shams and coworkers have identified circulating levels of anti-HSP27 antibody as a CVD risk factor in patients with chest pain and have also demonstrated significant interactions of the antibody with age in hypertension and hyperlipidemia.

Protein aggregation is a hallmark of cardiac stress conditions. One of the early reports on the stress response has shown that the vasculature is targeted upon stress and vascular heat shock protein response to stress arose from HSP70 induction. Also, the vasculature revealed differential regulation with coexpression of HSP27. In cardiac tissues, ischemic preconditioning (Chapter I, unit 1.3), is a protective function of cells to combat ischemic stress by an earlier ischemic episode that had resulted in a rapid induction of HSPs. Thereby, HSP induction is a gain-of-function of cardiomyocytes that eventually lead to cardioprotection by post-ischemic functional recovery. There exists a large number of literature on the protection of myocardial I/R injury by HSPs, especially HSP70 that reduce the infarct size and normalize cardiac function. Preinduction of HSP70 has been observed to protect cardiovascular functions after trauma-hemorrhage and resustication. Classic preconditioning offers potent protection and is however, short-lived. Delayed preconditioning is manifested subacutely around 24 h following preconditioning and offers protection against other ischemic pathologies. This type of second window preconditioning can be induced by pharmacological manipulations, endotoxins, exercise and heat stress. HSP72 confers tissue tolerance to I/R injury and an increase in HSP72 mRNA is concomitant with a qualitative increase in protein immunoreactivity. The small HSP, HSP27 is also fundamental to ischemia-induced delayed myocardial protection. The cardioprotective mechanisms of HSPs involve the inhibition of mitochondrial caspase-9 pathway of apoptosis by HSP27, HSP90 and HSP70. HSP27 protects the integrity of the microtubules and actin cytoskeleton in cardiac myocytes and endothelial cells exposed to ischemia. HSP90 binds to endothelial nitric oxide synthase (eNOS) and stimulates its activity. HSP70 enhances NO production in response to cytokine stimulation. Mild hyperthermic stress increases mitochondrial respiratory enzyme activity affording protection to mitochondrial energetics during prolonged cardiac preservation for transplantation. Integrated mitochondrial function is therefore protected against I/R injury in hyperthermia. HSP70 level has been identified as a marker for longevity in centenarian offsprings that avoid and/or delay cardiovascular diseases. Molecular chaperones are essential constituents of the cardiomyocytes. The αB-crystallin is a stress protein belonging to small HSP family that is associated with the muscle intermediate filaments and exerts its chaperoning functions in a polymerized form. A missense mutation of this gene, R120G is related to the familial desmin-related myopathy. αB-crystallin is constitutively and inducibly expressed and is the most abundant small HSP in the heart expressed in cardiomyocytes.

It has been studied that Ser-phosphorylation negatively regulates the chaperone function of αB-crystallin and cytoprotection is declined. Overexpression of HSPs differentially modulates protein kinase C (PKC) expression in neonatal cardiomyocytes. Therefore, it has been suggested that PKC may directly play a role in HSP-mediated cardioprotection. The mechanism by which PKC renders cardioprotection may be by HSP autoregulation. PKC may lead to phosphorylation of HSF1 and subsequently modulate HSP expression. In correlation, HSP overexpression has a direct effect on differential expression of the PKC isoforms. Another report by Heads and coworkers substantiates the differential cytoprotection in heat stress or hypoxia by the activation of stress protein genes in myogenic cells of embryonal rat hearts. Gender-specific differences in the incidence of cardiovascular diseases seem to be a specific area of interest. Though aged status is a cardiovascular risk factor, aged women are lesser susceptible and tolerant to CVDs. Estrogen therapy increases HSP72 levels in human coronary artery endothelial cells and also stimulates HSP90 mediated regulation of NO release.

Another important contribution to gender disparity of CVD has been elucidated by Knowlton and Sun in 2001 suggesting a mechanism for the heat shock protein expression in the heart. The activation of heat shock factor-1 (HSF-1) by steroid hormones (17β-estradiol and progesterone) resulting from a change in the interaction of HSP90 and HSF-1 represents a novel pathway in the upregulation of heat shock protein expression. HSPs are therefore extensively involved in cardioprotection mechanisms and contribute towards cardiomyocyte cytoprotection in the heart.

4.2. Association with Cellular ATP

Adenosine triphosphate (ATP) is the high energy source of cellular machinery. Energy-driven cellular mechanisms acquire high energy phosphates from ATP for metabolic turnover of the cell. Any depletion of ATP occurs in metabolic stress and we describe here the effects of ATP depletion as a cause and the consequence of heat shock protein response.

4.2.1. Effects of HSP70 on Cellular ATP-Depletion

In vivo, severe ATP depletion leads to proteotoxic stress resulting in dysfunction, destabilization and aggregation of cellular proteins. Sustained lack of ATP impairs cellular functions with subsequent cytotoxicity.

It has been observed that heat and metabolic preconditioning elevate intracellular HSP70 levels and reduce cell death after sustained ATP depletion without affecting the rate and extent of ATP decrease. Transient overexpression of HSP70 was shown to attenuate both cytotoxic and proteotoxic effects of ATP depletion. Excess HSP70 diminish ATP depletion-induced protein aggregation in the cytoplasm and nucleus. HSP70 accumulation mediates attenuation of proteotoxicity by elevated cell resistance to prolonged energy deprivation by improved formation of nonaggregable or soluble complexes between excess HSP70 and instable or damaged proteins in the cytosol and nucleosol. Thereby, HSP70-overexpressing cells preserve cellular proteins from ATP depletion-induced aggregation leading to cell death.

4.2.2. Effects of Cellular ATP Depletion on HSP90

HSP90 is constitutively expressed for the expression of many client proteins involved in cellular growth regulation. HSP90 is known to bind to ATP with ten-fold lower affinity than ADP and is therefore described as an 'ATP sensor' in the regulation of intracellular growth signaling cascades. Any ATP-depletion causes metabolic stress and results in disruption/dissociation of HSP90 from its client proteins and triggers rapid degradation of the proteins involved in cell growth that leads to activation of stress response. Hence, it is proposed that HSP90 chaperone plays a significant role in regulation of tissue growth both physiologically and pathologically. Thereby, the ATP-sensing activity of HSP90 explains the plausible mechanism by which metabolically stressed myocytes (cardiomyocytes) respond and regulate exogenous growth factor stimulation.

4.3. Mechanisms of Cardioprotection

Heat shock proteins play a central role in protection of the myocardium. Several mechanisms that mediate cardioprotection have been proposed and we describe here some of the main features of HSPs to regulate the attenuation of proteotoxicity and subsequent cytotoxicity in cardiac stress.

4.3.1. Chaperoning Functions

This is one of the primary functions of HSPs to restore cellular function. During cardiovascular stresses such as ischemia and reperfusion injury, accumulation of unfolded proteins and aggregation of these unfolded proteins occur leading to loss of cell viability. The ability to handle such stress conditions is offered by HSPs which are produced by a rapid transcription mechanism upon induction and are negatively regulated by means of an autoregulatory loop. Protein denaturation results from loss of native structural conformation which expose hydrophobic stretches. HSPs are targeted towards these hydrophobic regions and the amendment of native protein structure is effected. Structural disruption of the cell and subsequent necrosis is therefore prevented.

4.3.2. Preservation of ATP

Depletion of cellular ATP is detrimental to the cell effecting protein aggregation, breakdown of cytoskeleton and loss of ionic balance. It has been demonstrated earlier that HSPs respond to ATP-depletion and exhibit ATP-sparing effects. Induction of HSPs in cardioplegic arrest and reperfusion has resulted in beneficial changes in the high energy phosphate metabolism. Cardioprotective effects of HSP70 have been shown to elevate ATP and phosphocreatinine levels following ischemia. The protective effects of HSPs in energy preservation have been shown to be due to a reduction in purine catabolite release and an improved functional recovery.

4.3.3. Activation of Potassium Channels

It has been observed that heat shock protein response in ischemic preconditioning has been associated with opening of ATP-sensitive potassium channels (K_{ATP}). This has not yet been identified as due to the stress or the stress proteins but potassium channel inhibitor studies have shown a blockade of reduction in infarct size, a characteristic function of HSPs.

4.3.4. Inhibition of Apoptosis

Apoptosis has earlier been described in Chapter II, Unit 2.6. HSPs act to inhibit the apoptotic pathway during cardiovascular stress, under conditions of which apoptotic cell death is averted. HSP70 and HSP27 have shown to be potent regulators of apoptosis in ischemic injury and heat stress. Thereby, HSPs mediate cardioprotection by an antiapoptotic function.

4.4. HSP-Mediated Protection in Cardiovascular Stress

Molecular chaperones are essential components of the cardiomyocytes, constitutively expressed in minimal levels for normal cardiac function and are raised in terms of inducible expression in response to cardiac stress.

The loss-of-function of the HSPs compromises the ability to handle stress while HSP gain-of-function offers cardioprotection. CVDs upregulate an array of HSPs for eventual cardioprotection, thereby, requiring further insights of the potential roles of HSP response.

4.4.1. Myocardial Infarction

Tissue damage from myocardial infarction (MI) occurs as a result of the initial ischemic event and subsequent injury resulting from reperfusion. Ischemic preconditioning against subsequent sustained ischemia and reperfusion (I/R injury) is an inherent ability of the myocardium to prevent subsequent ischemic damage. Preconditioning involves a cascade of stress signals such as activation of protein kinase C (PKC) , protein tyrosine kinases (PTKs) and mitogen-activated protein kinases (MAPKs).

These kinase modulations effect the opening of K_{ATP} channels, upregulation of nitric oxide synthase (NOS), induction of cyclooxygenase-2 (COX-2), cellular antioxidants and a dramatically increased expression of a number of protective proteins known as the heat shock proteins. Ischemic preconditioning elicit the synthesis of major HSPs in the heart. A possible S-O-S factor maybe due to phosphorylation of proteins via PKC activation to effect cardioprotection.

HSP70 may counteract important mechanisms of ischemic injury including unfolding, misfolding or pathological modification of critical proteins. It is hypothesized that circulating HSP70 may correlate with the extent of myocardial damage in acute myocardial infarction (AMI). HSP70 concentration is related to the size of the infarction, and, is therefore a potent marker of myocardial damage. HSP72, an inducible form of the HSP70 family, is strongly induced in the myocardium under stress conditions of acute cardiac overload and ischemia. HSP72 plays a pivotal role in protection of cells from subsequent myocardial injury. HSP90 aids in the modulation of cytoskeletal dynamics of the stressed cells to attain myocardial protection.

An ischemic condition is a potent inducer of HSP60. Small heat shock proteins also act to preventcardiac dysfunction which will be discussed in Section 4.4.6. Gray and his coworkers (1999) have proposed that heat stress preconditioning was beneficial for ischemic myocardium.

4.4.2. Heart Failure

Diverse changes in the production of myocardial HSPs occur during development of chronic heart failure. Significant alterations of HSP27, HSP60 and HSP72 occur. These disparate patterns of HSPs during end-stage failing human hearts with ischemic or dilated cardiomyopathy have been documented by Knowlton and coworkers. It is difficult to determine whether an alteration in HSP levels of the human failing heart can be attributed to heart failure following due to hypertension, hyperlipidemia and atherosclerosis. Exposure to heat shock and I/R injury increases HSP27 and HSP72 in cardiomyocytes. Levels of HSP27 and HSP72 with no marked increase during the progression of heart failure at 8th week suggests that the failing heart may attenuate the ability to produce the two HSPs.Apoptotic death of cardiomyocytes is enhanced in the failing heart. HSP70 reduces myocardial apoptotic cell death. An increase in HSP60 at 8th week and its location in the mitochondria reflect that mitochondria are exposed to unknown stress at the decompensatory stage of chronic heart failure, with a lowered mitochondrial function of the viable left ventricle, accompanied by a significant reduction in the level of high energy phosphates. A study of HSP72 in the right heart failure indicated its induction in the heart and liver but not in lungs and peripheral muscles representing an intracellular marker of stress reaction that can persist chronically. The presence of chronic heart failure seems to specifically influence the cardiac HSP72 gene and the activation of sympathetic system. HSP72 does not play a protective role against the development of chronic heart failure, but in analogy with the neuroendocrine response, HSP expression in the affected organs represents an unsuccessful form of intracellular adaptation to the new condition. Probably, HSP overexpression counteracts the deleterious effects of oxygen free radicals or by chaperoning protein folding, preventing the formation of protein aggregation with an increase in protein turnover in chronic heart failure. Levels of HSP60 double in end-stage heart failure. The inflammatory state of heart failure cause translocation of HSP60 to the plasma membrane and this provides a pathway for cardiac injury. Localization of HSP60 to cell surface correlates with increased apoptosis. In heart failure, HSP60 is present in plasma membrane, on the cell surface and in the plasma. Therefore, it is postulated that abnormal trafficking of HSP60 to the cell surface is an early tigger for myocyte loss and progression to heart failure. The purpose of our book aims at the cardioprotection offered by HSPs, but the effects of HSP60 in augmentation of CVD is provided with reference to the intriguing roles of HSP60 as well.

4.4.3. Hypertension

Hypertension occurs as a result of osmotic imbalance due to an impaired rening-angiotensin system. An osmotic stress protein, OSP94 has been identified in mouse renal medullary cells, which is regulated by a hypertonicity-sensitive *cis*-acting element OSP94-TonE which is distinct from the heat shock element (HSE). Recently, the authors have identified OSP94 protein in hypertensive human heart. OSP94 is induced in response to the osmotic imbalance prevalent in hypertensive tissues. OSP94 is known to possess an ATP-binding N-terminal region similar to other ATP-binding HSPs. OSP94 is a member of the HSP110 family due to its sequence similarity. It is also inducible by heat shock, however, its subcellular location has not yet been identified. The major function of OSP94 is to act as a molecular chaperone and participates in the UPR. It is a homodimeric protein and additionally, has a nucleotide-binding function.

The circulating levels of HSP60 in borderline hypertension become elevated. It could therefore be involved in induction/progression of hypertension accounted by its proinflammatory function and hence, serve as markers for early cardiovascular disease.

Raised blood pressure has direct effects on the vasculature and vessels subjected to greater mechanical and shear stress express express heat shock proteins. HSP70 mRNA levels are enhanced in hypertensive elements and there is greater accumulation of heat stress-induced HSP70 mRNA in peripheral blood lymphocytes from hypertensive humans. This phenomenon demonstrates a stress response to hypertension. The stress response of HSP release protects neighbouring cells and HSP70 enhances the survival of stressed cultured arterial smooth muscle cells. Heat shock protein expression is secondary to the inflammatory process. The expression of cytokines by both the vascular endothelium and infiltrating leukocyte population drives the expression or release of heat shock proteins from the vessel wall. A spectrum of inflammatory cytokines such as interferon-γ, interleukin-1α and -1β and tumor necrosis factor-α (TNF-α) increases the HSP expression in a range of cell types. Alternatively, the localized expression of heat shock proteins may also promote the production of cytokines, the enhanced expression of adhesion molecules and the establishment and propagation of the inflammatory response. A prior heat shock treatment induces a greater elevation of HSP70 and HSP27 expression in angiotensin II (Ang-II)-induced hypertension and correlate the interaction of HSPs and the nuclear factor-κB (NF-κB) pathway. HSP70 and HSP27 peaked at 24h, higher above basal levels, associated with suppression of Ang II-induced hypertension, NF-κB activation and interleukin IL-6 expression, enhancing postischemic myocardial recovery. The cardioprotection of HSP70 and HSP27 are attributed to their functions to act as molecular chaperones by regulation of refolding and renaturation of damaged proteins. They interact with smooth muscle proteins such as AT1 receptor to regulate the tone of blood vessels. Heat shock treatment modulates endothelium-dependent vascular relaxation by the anti-oxygen free radical role of HSPs. HSPs also block apoptotic signaling pathways exhibiting anti-apoptotic function. HSPs sense conformational changes of the inhibitor I-κB protein, perform their chaperoning functions and interact with modified I-κB to prevent subsequent phosphorylation, degradation and dissociation from NF-κB complexes promoting NF-κB-mediated antiapoptosis.

4.4.4. Hypoxia

HSP60 is a targeted chaperone in hypoxia. HSP60 is found primarily in mitochondria, and 15-20% is found in the cytosol. HSP60 complexes with Bax in the cytosol and any reduction in HSP60 lead to translocation of Bax to the mitochondria and trigger apoptosis. In hypoxia, disassociation of HSP60-Bax complex results in translocation of cytosolic HSP60 to the plasma membrane and addition of Bax to the mitochondria releases cytochrome c and subsequent caspase activation further leading to apoptosis. These changes occur before reoxygenation and the concomitant generation of free-radicals. This suggests that HSP60 has a regulatory role for the activity of proapoptotic proteins and is a key antiapoptotic protein in the cell. It is also suggested that HSP60 may have membrane-stabilizing properties.

4.4.5. Atrial Fibrillation

Atrial HSPs are increased in clinical atrial fibrillation (AF) and this response correlates with reduced AF perpetuation. Higher levels of HSP expression are associated with a decreased risk of postoperative AF. HSPs have potentially significant antioxidant properties and there is evidence that oxidant stress contributes to the pathophysiology of AF. Thus, prevention of oxidant-stress injury is a potential contributor to HSP-mdediated protection against tachycardia remodeling and associated AF promotion. Thereby, HSP induction protects against AF. Upregulation of HSP60, HSP10, and HSP75 (a mitochondrial member of the HSP70 family) expression in chronic AF has been observed. Factors that have been shown to increase HSPs in the heart include tumor necrosis factor TNF-α, stretch and decreased shortening. A 2.5 times increase of HSP60 levels has been reported in chronic AF. Chronic stimulation of cardiac myocytes with TNF-α lead to an initial increase in HSP72 levels, however, the myocytes become desensitized within 24h and the levels of HSP72 return to basal values and this is true for AF hearts as well. HSC73 maybe associated with different stages of AF. The expression of HSP60 might be associated with the degree of atrial mylosis. It remains to be determined why HSPs have differential expression levels during different stages of AF and whether the HSPs play any role in the pathogenesis of AF and in mylosis.

4.4.6. Small Heat Shock Proteins in Cardioprotection

The small HSP subfamily also represents one of the best studied stress proteins. In earlier studies, Lam et al. in 1996, have isolated and characterized cDNA of human heart encoding HSPL27, a novel member of sHSPs, named 27 kDa heat shock protein-like protein. Another new member of the sHSP family was identified as HSPB2, with a genomic locus less than 1 kb from the 5'-end of the αB-crystallin gene with opposite transcription direction. It is also reported that HSPB2 gene was expressed preferentially in skeletal muscle and heart. In mammalian species, sHSPs comprise of: HSP27, HSPB1, HSPB2, HSPB3, αA-crystallin (HSPB4), αB-crystallin (HSPB5), HSP25, HSP20 (HSPB6), HSPB7, HSP22 (HSPB8), HSPB9 and HSPB10. The sHSPs have been classified into two main categories: Classes I and II, according to their different patterns of gene expression and subcellular localization. All sHSPs share a common α-crystallindomain with unique N-terminal and C-terminal extensions and the latter is critical for their chaperone activity.

HSP27 is fundamental to ischemia-induced delayed myocardial protection. I/R injury also induces overexpression of HSP27 which acts to substantiate cardioprotection after repetitive insults. Earlier studies have well demonstrated the cardioprotective roles of HSP27 in isolated hearts *in vitro*. HSP27 is constitutively expressed in all eukaryotic cells and also induced upon heat stress with a highly conserved α-crystallin domain. Kwon and team have reported the potential cytoprotective effects of HSP27 as a therapeutic protein in cardiomyocytes using a protein delivery system. HSP27 displays cytoprotectivity during I/R injury by significantly reducing the infarct size. A possible mechanism by which HSP27 protects against cell death can be explained by its interaction with Akt performing a chaperone function by maintaining the kinase in a biologically active conformation, which directs the cell to choose an antiapoptotic course. HSP27 phosphorylation is essential to suppress atrial tachycardia remodeling. Phosphorylated HSP27 isoforms stabilize actin filaments and prevent their remodeling. It is also reported that expression of HSP27 is correlated to cell survival of cardiomyocytes in response to apoptotic stimuli. This protectivity could be attributed to the direct inhibition of caspase cascade activation to inhibit apoptosis. Wang et al. in 2007, have identified that ATF5 (activating transcription factor 5) could promote cell survival and increase cell tolerance of the cardiomyocytes. HSP27 is also shown to be cardioprotective in offering resistance to doxorubicin (Dox)-induced cardiac dysfunction. Subsequently, following Dox administration, HSP27 was found to be elevated and played a critical role in improving left ventricular (LV) systolic and diastolic functions by suppressing oxidative status and apoptosis. Thus, HSP27 is a key heat shock protein molecule in cardioprotection under stress or Dox-induced cardiac stress. HSP25, another member of the sHSP seems to be involved in cardiomyocyte differentiation. HSP20 is a molecular chaperone which functions to assist proteins in achieving and maintaining proper conformation. HSP20 enhances cardiac function and renders cardiac protection against β-agonist-mediated apoptosis and I/R injury. HSP20 has also been linked to calcium handling. Cardiomyocyte permeabilization with HSP20 results in a significant increase in cell shortening and a decrease in calcium transient values. Additionally, HSP20 increases the amplitudes of both calcium transients and cell contraction in cardiomyocytes. Recently, Islamovic and coworkers have investigated the C-terminal extension of HSP20 to provide a mechanistic insight into itspossible function. I/R injury resulted in cardioprotection by HSP20 only by overexpression of fulllength HSP20, while substitution of its C-terminal did not show any protectivity. HSP20 binds to actin in vitro and in vivo and the association with actin is dependent on the phosphorylation state of HSP20. Phosphorylated HSP20 associates with globular actin, whereas nonphosphorylated HSP20 associates with filamentous actin, thereby enhancing myocardial contraction. HSP20 directly interacts with the proapoptotic protein Bax. This suggests that the cardioprotective mechanisms of HSP20 may be mediated through prevention of the translocation of Bax from the cytosol into the mitochondrion, which leads to the restriction of cytochrome c release and repression of caspase-3 activation.

HSP32 [Heme oxygenase-1 (HO-1)] is a unique protein (acting on heme) and is induced in response to oxidative stress. HSP32 acts as a mediator of cytoprotection in ischemic heart disease, delayed myocardial preconditioning and cardiovascular damage by inhibition of oxidative stress and offers cellular protection. Phosphorylation by activation of protein kinases and hypoxia has also been reported to induce HSP32 in cardiomyocytes. HSP32 plays a cytoprotective role and exerts anti-inflammatory, antiapoptotic, antioxidant effects, and is also recently known to possess proangiogenic properties. In a recent study, HSP32 has been reported to inhibit postmyocardial infarct remodeling and influence the restoration of ventricular function.

4.4.7. Heat Shock Proteins in Cardiac Pathophysiologies

Cardiac stress also results from various pathophysiological factors eliciting a number of stress proteins. Snoeckx et al (2001) have described important relations of these pathological insults of the cardiac tissues and the strategic responses of HSPs. An important factor in considering the potential of HSPs to improve cardiac function during and after ischemia is the age of the tissues under investigation. Tissue aging seems to increase susceptibility to cardiac ischemia in aged humans. It is known that overall gene transcription, mRNA translation, and protein degradation were decreased during senescence, whereas a number of malfunctioning proteins were increased. Because HSP-mediated stress protection could be of special interest in aged individuals, several studies have been initiated to evaluate their potential in this population group. The stress-induced synthesis of HSPs was reduced in the aging cardiovascular system and cardiac HSP70 synthesis upon heat shock was substantially lower than in young rats. It may be concluded that the heat shock response is reduced in aged hearts and limited HSP synthesis showed reduced protective effects on ischemia tolerance.

Pathological myocardial hypertrophy is acknowledged to be a major risk factor for, myocardial infarction and heart failure. The pathologically hypertrophied heart is more susceptible to ischemic damage. Sustained poor cardiac output, permanent arrhythmias, and increased loss of intracellular enzymes are commonly observed during postischemic reperfusionof hypertrophied hearts. This poor function is often associated with myocardial contracture and asubstantial underperfusion of subendocardial layers of the left ventricular wall.

Understanding the potential of hypertrophied cardiac tissue to upregulate HSP synthesis would be highly valuable, since these proteins could attenuate the poor ischemia tolerance in this type of heart. HSP70 and HSP60 were transiently overexpressed, while low levels of HSP90 were observed. Induction of HSPs in tissues to be transplanted is still under investigations, although available reports are scarce. Heat pretreatment of a longlasting hypothermic storage of cardiac tissue resulted in a signifi cantly improved and accelerated recovery of developed pressure and coronary flow, while the residual ATP and total energy-rich phosphate tissue content was signifi cantly higher than in non-retreated control hearts. HSP70 tissue content has been used as a marker for the risk of rejection of tissue transplants. In transplanted tissues, high HSP levels reflect a response to inflammation, apoptosis, and/or necrosis.

4.5. Proteomics of HSP Response

The development of proteomics since 1995, has prompted researchers to investigate its potential application in cardiovascular research. There has been a striking surge of interest for proteomic analysis in cardiovascular biology in view of its current thrust (Arrel et al. 2001; Jiang et al. 2001; Macri and Rapundalo, 2001; McGregor and Dunn, 2003; Borozdenkova et al. 2004; Dohke et al. 2006; Doll et al. 2007).

Changes to the cardiovascular system arise from or have the potential to alter, proteomes of cardiac muscle and components of the vascular system, including smooth muscle and endothelial cells. Such changes may be documented through an integrated series of proteomic approaches. A detailed 2-DE analysis of dilated cardiomyopathy-diseased human myocardial tissue revealed more than fifty HSP27 protein species by immunoblotting. Protein changes of HSP72, HSP70i, mitochondrial HSP70 precursor, mitochondrial stress protein (HSP70-related), HSP60, mitochondrial matrix protein p1 (membrane-bound HSP60), αB-crystallin and HSP27 have been documented by proteomic analysis in cardiovascular diseases.

The causes of cardiac dysfunction likely result from alternations in cardiac protein expression. Therefore, determining the posttranslational modifications of cardiac proteins in response to cardiomyopathies is important to provide unique insights and an understanding of the mechanisms of cardiac malfunctions. Dohke et al. (2006) have performed the proteomic analysis of cardiac sHSP expression in congestive heart failure (CHF). It was observed that the cardiac sHSPs were highly expressed after the induction of CHF. The increased expression of αB-crystallin and HSP27 decreased serum markers of cardiac damage against hypoxic myocardial injury. HSP20 was significantly increased in CHF compared to the normal heart. It is therefore evident that three cardiac sHSPs, namely, HSP20, HSP27 and αB-crystallin play a critical compensatory role in the pathophysiology of CHF.

4.6. Regulation of HSP Expression by Signaling Mechanisms

Heat shock proteins are mostly inducible and several pathways co-exist for the induction of HSPs. Identification of signaling pathways for induction of HSPs rely on various cellular components and is still a poorly understood phenomenon. Kacimi et al. (2000) have investigated the role of kinases in hypoxia-induced HSP expression and their plausible effects on HSP induction. The kinases that contribute to the induction of HSPs include protein kinase C and the mitogen-activated protein kinase family (MAPK), that comprise of extracellular-signal regulated kinase (ERK), c-Jun NH_2-terminal kinase and the stress-activated protein kinase (JNK/SAPK) and p38. Hypoxia leads to activation of multiple kinase cascades in the cardiomyocytes. p38 stress kinase appears to play a direct role in the regulation of HSP32 expression. In contrast, HSP70 is strongly affected by the multiple kinase cascade signaling. Hypoxia induced phosphorylation of MAPKAP-2/3 activated kinases and HSP27 by the activation of signaling pathways downstream of p38 stress kinase. Phosphorylation on Ser residues mediated by stress kinase modulates the activity of HSP27. Phosphorylation of HSP27 is an important post-translational modification in cultured cardiac myocytes in response to hypoxia, and plays a significant role in cardioprotection. Thereby a differential pattern of regulation of HSPs has been observed by the kinase cascade signaling mechanisms. The regulation of heat shock response is mediated by cytosolic proteins known as heat shock factors (HSF) that interact with a specific regulatory element, the heat shock element (HSE) in the promoter region of the HSP gene. HSF activation is one of the earliest responses observed in many different cells exposed to stresses, such as ischemia, hypoxia, hyperthermia and mechanical stretch. Stretch is a common phenomenon in both the normal and diseased cardiovascular system. Increased stretch occurs with hypertension, heart failure and myocardial infarction. Stretch-activated ion channels (SACs) may act as mechanotransducers to mediate stress-induced gene expression and is an important signaling pathway in induction of stress response. Mechanical stretch and isovolumic contraction are sufficient to initiate the heat shock response without neural and humoral factors. Activation of stretch-dependent channels results in cation influx, which is associated with gene expression and protein synthesis. A dual-function cochaperone/ubiquitin ligase, CHIP (carboxyl terminus of HSP70-interacting protein) is highly expressed in the heart and regulates chaperone activity and protein quality control. It interacts with HSP70 and enhances refolding of stress-damaged proteins *in vivo* and is therefore required for maximal cardioprotection after myocardial infarction thereby coordinating the response to cardiac stress. Cardiac cells respond to extracellular stimuli by activating signal transduction cascades, largely involving protein kinases. We shall discuss the regulation of cardiac stress by the action of protein kinases and their signaling pathways.

4.6.1. Regulation of HSP Response by MAPK Signaling Pathways

MAPKs are an important group of signal-transducing protein kinases which act by phosphorylating various substrates including transcription factors which regulate the expression of specific sets of genes and hence can mediate specific genetic responses to extracellular stimuli. MAPKs consist of three levels in signal transduction: MAPK kinase kinase (MKKK) which activates a MAPK kinase (MKK) which finally activates the MAPK. These three-kinase cascades are organized in modules which are conserved from yeast to humans reflecting their physiological importance throughout phylogenesis. MAPK require both Tyr and Thr phosphorylation to become activated. Tyr and Thr phosphorylation of MAPK results from dual specificity kinases. The Ser/Thr kinase MKKK phosphorylates a dual-specificity kinase MKK which phosphorylates a Thr-X-Thr motif in the activation loop of a MAPK. MAPK are proline-directed protein kinases. The vast majority of their identified substrates are transcription factors, but other nuclear substrates, cytosolic and structural proteins can also be phosphorylated by MAPK. The phosphorylation of transcription factors by MAPK can occur via three distinct pathways. Firstly, activated MAPKcan translocate from the cytoplasm to the nucleus and phosphorylate transcription factors there. Second, MAPK can phosphorylate transcription factors in the cytosol and the phosphorylated transcription factors then translocate to the nucleus. Third, MAPK can activate other protein kinases which then directly or indirectly act on transcription factors, either in the cytosol or in the nucleus. MAPK play a potential role as mediators of injury and/or protection in myocardial ischemia, reperfusion, ischemic preconditioning and hypertrophy and are apparent regulators of cardiac function.

4.6.2. Regulation of HSP Induction by Ras/Rac Pathways

Small GTP-binding proteins Ras and Rac are activated by cyclic strain stress, which mediate MAPK phosphatase-1 expression. Increases in the elongational and transitional mobility in cell membranes activate membrane-bound G proteins by facilitating exchange of GDP to GTP, subsequently leading to HSF1 activation and HSP70 expression. Ras has 3 major effectors, namely the Raf Ser and Thr protein kinases that act upstream of ERKs, lipid and protein kinase phosphatidylinositol 3-kinase (P13K), and Ral-GDS, a guanine-nucleotide (GEF) exchange factor for the small G protein Ral. Ras can activate Rac through P13K. Rac, inturn activates the p21-activated protein kinases (PAKs), which are known to induce JNK/SAPK and p38 activation. The signaling pathway regulating HSP70 expression by cyclic strain stress is:

Ras ⟶ P13K ⟶ Rac ⟶ PAK ⟶ ? ⟶ HSF1 ⟶ HSP70 transcription

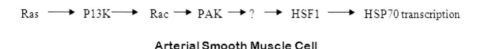

Arterial Smooth Muscle Cell

Figure 4.1. Regulation of HSP70 expression.

Thus Rac and Ras seem to be required for cyclic strain stress-induced HSF1 activation in a manner independent of extracellular signal-regulated protein kinase (ERK) and p38 MAPK.

4.6.3. Regulation of HSP Expression by JAK-STAT Pathways

The growh-stimulating effects of thrombin are mediated primarily via activation of a G protein-coupled receptor, protease-activated receptor PAR1. PAR1 has no intrinsic Tyr kinase activity, yet requires Tyr phosphorylation events to induce mitogenesis.

Janus tyrosine kinases (JAKs) are one of the 11 mammalian non-receptor Tyr kinase families that were initially identified as essential mediators of cellular signaling induced by the interactions of cytokines with their cognate receptors. There are 4 members of the JAK family, JAK1, JAK2, JAK3 and TYK2. JAKs are essential for cytokine-induced signaling.

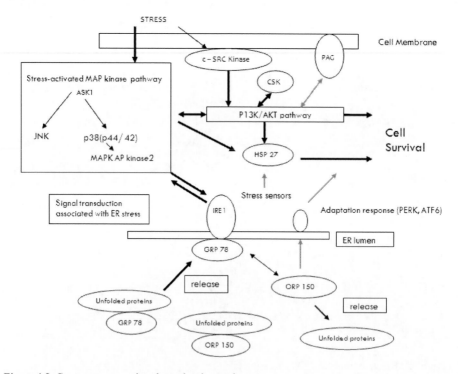

Figure 4.2. Stress response signal tranduction pathway.

Investigations of the roles of JAKs in thrombin-mediated signaling show that JAK2 was activated in vascular smooth muscle cells (VSMC) treated with thrombin and signal transducers and activators of transcription (STAT1 and STAT3) were phosphorylated and translocated to the nucleus in a JAK2-dependent manner. JAK2 is present upstream of Ras in the Ras/Raf/MEK/ERK pathway and thus implicate JAK2 in regulation of early growth esponse genes and cell proliferation.

JAK-STAT pathway by thrombin is via the generation of intracellular Reactive oxygen species (ROS), the cellular effects of which are modulated by HSPs. Therefore, thrombin might induce HSP expression in VSMC, documented by the presence of functional STAT-binding sites in HSP70 and HSP90 promoters, suggesting that HSP synthesis is regulated via the JAK-STAT pathway. Thus, JAK-STAT pathway activation is necessary for thrombin-induced VSMC growth and HSP gene expression. ROSsuch as H2O2 activate intracellular signal transduction pathways implicated in the pathogenesis of CVDs. It has been observed that JAK2 was rapidly activated in VSMCs treated with H_2O_2 and STAT1 and STAT3 were Tyr-phosphorylated and translocated to the nucleus in a JAK2-dependent manner. H_2O_2 stimulated HSP70 expression in a time-dependent manner. H_2O_2 activated HSP70 promoter via enhanced binding of STATs to cognate binding sites in the promoter. Thus, regulation of HSP70 chaperone is via activation of JAK/STAT pathway which help VSMCs adapt to oxidative stress.

4.6.4. Associated Signaling Pathways in Cardiac Stress

ROCK (Rho-associated kinase) pathway is implicated in cardiovascular aberrations and is detrimental to the heart. However, this pathway has no direct role on HSPs, but inhibition of this pathway activates the endothelial nitric oxide synthase (eNOS) which has a protective effect on the vasculature. ROCK activity is involved in the expression of plasminogen activator inhibitor-1 (PAI-1) mediated by hyperglycemia, indicating that the RhoA/ROCK pathway may be beneficial in CVD and could be a potential therapeutic target. Specifically, the RhoA/ROCK pathway has been shown to be involved in angiogenesis, atherosclerosis, hypertension, myocardial hypertrophy, myocardial I/R injury and vascular remodeling. Any defect in the pathways of induction of HSPs may lead to deprivation of the protective mechanisms following cardiac stress and eventually lead to apoptosis and increase the potency of cardiovascular risks. Therefore, strategies requiring the modulation of HSP pathways are still to be investigated, also for exploitation of therapeutic measures in cardiac stress.

References

Arrell DK, Neverova I and Van Eyk JE (2001) Cardiovascular proteomics: evolution and potential. *Circ. Res.* 88: 763-773.

Bornfeldt KE (2000) Stressing Rac, Ras, and downstream heat shock protein 70. *Circ. Res.* 86: 1101-1103.

Borozdenkova S, Westbrook JA, Patel V, Wait R, Bolad I, Burke MM, Bell AD, Banner NR, Dunn MJand Rose ML (2004) Use of proteomics to discover novel markers of cardiac allograft rejection. *J.Proteome Res.*3: 282–288.

Chang J, Wasser JS, Cornelussen RNM and Knowlton AA (2001) Activation of heat shock factor by stretch-activated channels in rat hearts. *Circ.* 104: 209-214.

Dohke T, Wada A, Isono T, Fujii M, Yamamoto T, Tsutamoto Tand Horie M (2006) Proteomic analysis reveals aignificant alternations of cardiac small heat shock protein expression in congestive heart failure. *J.Card.Fail.* 12: 77-84.

Doll D, Sarikas A, Krajcik R and Zolk O (2007) Proteomic expression analysis of cardiomyocytes subjected to proteasome inhibition. *Biochem. Biophys. Res. Commun.* 353: 436-442.

Jiang L, Tsubakihara M, Heinke MY, Yao M, Dunn MJ, Phillips W, dos Remedios CG and Nosworthy NJ (2001) Heart failure and apoptosis: Electrophoretic methods support data from micro- and macro-arrays. A critical review of genomics and proteomics. *Proteomics* 1: 1481-1488.

Kacimi R, Chentoufi J, Honbo N, Long CS and Karliner JS (2000) Hypoxia differentially regulates stress proteins in cultured cardiomyocytes: role of the p38 stress-activated kinase signaling cascade, and relation to cytoprotection. *Cardiovasc. Res.* 46: 139-150.

Macri J and Rapundalo ST (2001) Application of proteomics to the study of cardiovascular biology. *Trends Cardiovasc. Med.* 11: 66-75.

Madamanchi NR, Li S, Patterson C and Runge MS (2001) Thrombin regulates vascular smooth muscle cell growth and heat shock proteins via the JAK-STAT pathway. *J. Biol. Chem.* 276: 18915-18924.

Mala JGS and Takeuchi S (2008) Heat shock proteins in cardiovascular stress. *Clin. Med. Insights: Cardiol.* 2: 245-256.

McGregor E and Dunn MJ (2003) Proteomics of heart disease. *Hum. Mol.Genet.* 12: R135-R144.

Michel MC, Li Y and Heusch G (2001) Mitogen-activated protein kinases in the heart. *Naunyn- Schmiedeberg's Arch. Pharmacol.* 363: 245-266.

Noma K, Oyama N and Liao JK (2006) Physiological role of ROCKs in the cardiovascular system. *Am. J Physiol. Cell Physiol.* 290: 661-668.

Xu Q, Schett G, Li C, Hu Y and Wick G (2000)Mechanical stress-induced heat shock protein 70 expression in vascular smooth muscle cells is regulated by Rac and Ras small G proteins but not mitogen-activated protein kinases. *Circ. Res.* 86: 1122-1128.

In: Heat Shock Proteins …
Authors: S. Takeuchi and J. G. S. Mala

ISBN: 978-1-61324-589-7
© 2012 Nova Science Publishers, Inc.

Chapter V

Heat Shock Proteins and Therapeutics

Abstract

Heat shock proteins display chaperoning properties to prevent protein denaturation and aggregation and inhibit apoptosis for cell survival. Targeting these proteins in cardiovascular ailments as therapeutics is a sustained effort in most laboratories. A lot of literature is available in the recent years on the use of HSPs as anti-cancer vaccines. However, their potency in treatment of vascular dysfunctions is still not completely understood. This Chapter is devoted to describe the essential roles of the HSPs to undertake prophylactic measures in the near future. An increase in HSP expression or induction of the HSP response is a validated criterion to treat heart ailments as well. Hence, drugs that induce HSP response can be an efficient means of therapeutic use. However, the pharmacological response of the drug may be unsafe in vivo and there exists a need for direct HSP therapy for safer therapeutics. We hereby discuss some available resources that implicate HSPs in cardioprotection.

5.1. Heat Shock Proteins in Cardiac Therapy

The heart has a remarkable capability to handle stress by 'ischemic preconditioning' from the induction of HSPs by an earlier mild stress to offer cardioprotection. This suggests that HSPs have the potential to play a therapeutic role in CVDs. This effect can be used to target the development of clinical procedures to elevate HSP expression in a safe and efficient manner using pharmacological or gene therapeutic strategies. It is of particular interest that elevated temperature induces HSP expression in the heart during transportation prior to cardiac transplantation and mild heat treatment before hypothermic storage enhances subsequent recovery of the heart. However, age is a considerable factor that promotes risk of impaired activation of HSF-1 by stress. This effect is also associated with a reduced protective response subjected to ischemic stress in aged hearts. Hence, there should be a striking balance between the severity and status of cardiac pathology and the therapeutic potential of HSPs. Protein transduction domain (PTD)-mediated delivery of HSP27 on I/R injury represents a potential therapeutic strategy for ischemic heart diseases. Thus, the promise of HSP-induced cardiac therapy can be classified into (1) Pharmacological method and (2) Gene therapy.

5.1.1. Pharmacological Method

Non-stressful inducers have also been shown to induce HSP synthesis. It has been demonstrated that interleukin-6-like cytokine cardiotrophin-1 (CT-1) induced HSP synthesis in cultured cardiac cells which protected against ischemic stress during subsequent exposure. Also, tyrosine kinase inhibitor herbimycin A induced such tolerance mechanisms. Bimoclomol (BM), a novel hydroxylamine derivative induced HSP synthesis in intact perfused heart ex vivo and produced protection against subsequent ischemia. Similarly, norepinephrine treatment induced cardioprotection against subsequent ischemic stress. Preconditioning by activation of adenosine A_1 receptors was accompanied by phosphorylation of HSP27 which enhanced carioprotection. However, it is of utmost importance that induction of HSPs should be attained without any consequences of side-effects. For example, CT-1 also induces cardiac hypertrophy, while herbimycin A also has a detrimental effect on cell growth and cell division. Induction of HSPs without eliciting a full stress response is on the keen interest and appears to be promising in the near future.

5.1.2 Gene Therapy

The risk potentials of induction of HSPs by stressful and pharmacological agents that cause side-effects could be reduced by a direct delivery of HSPs genes to the heart. HSP70 gene within a plasmid vector delivered directly to the heart via intra-coronary infusion of liposomal particles containing it conferred effective protection against subsequent ischemia or endotoxin-induced cardiac damage.

All the more, the problem of gene delivery to safely and efficiently deliver the gene to the target tissue without side-effects still remains unresolved. Use of viral vector-mediated gene delivery and modeling of liposomes is a valid approach to investigate the importance of HSP therapy especially in human systems.

Thus, the challenge is to identify pharmacological/gene therapy to elevate HSP levels in the intact heart without succumbing to undesired side-effects and without stressful procedures is in the line of investigation in the present status.

5.2. Targeting HSP Expression in Atrial Fibrillation

Drugs that boost endogenous HSP response have been of particular interests in atrial fibrillation (AF). Pharmacological approaches to prevent atrial remodeling have been on the rise. Drugs with T-type Ca^{2+} channel blocking action such as mibefradil and amiodarone prevent atrial tachycardia remodeling.

Interventions with antiinflammatory and/or antioxidant actions such as glucocorticoids and statins prevent atrial remodeling by induction of HSPB1 (HSP27)expression and phosphorylation by the co-induction property of HSPB1 (HSP27)which represents a novel anti-remodeling intervention in AF. Geranylgeranylacetone (GGA) is a drug often used for boosting HSP expression that induces HSP synthesis in various tissues by activation of the heat shock transcription factor HSF1. HSP induction by GGA treatment attenuates atrial structural remodeling and AF promotion in canine models of CHF and acute ischemia-induced AF. The protective effects of GGA against AF-related atrial remodeling suggest the potential therapeutic value of inducers of heat shock response as well.

5.3. Pharmacological Modulation of HSP Response

An antifungal antibiotic, radicicol is known to induce heat shock response in neonatal rat cardiomyocytes by its ability to activate HSF1-HSE complex formation. It displays a binding effect on HSP90 and is directly dependent on the amount of HSP90 present in the cell, thereby protecting against I/R injury in cardiomyocytes.

Radicicol-induced HSP increase has significant consequences by imparting cardioprotection in subsequent I/R injury. Binding of radicicol to the amino-terminal ATP site of HSP90 render the HSP90 nonfunctional, whereas it does not reduce the HSP90 cellular level, thus exhibiting a novel therapeutic role in the treatment of cardiac I/R injury.

5.4. Membrane-Lipid Therapy of Stress Protein Response

Bimoclomol is a potent inducer of heat shock response and has therapeutic implications in treatment of heart diseases. The effets of BM on HSP co-expression are mediated via HSF1 activation, which shows enhanced nuclear transport and binding to DNA. It is of significant observation that, BM does not affect protein denaturation but exhibits specific effects on membrane lipids and modifies membrane domains upon a sense of stress and causes enhanced activation of HSP genes. This is termed 'membrane-lipid therapy' in which drugs that influence lipid organization induce a concomitant modulation of membrane-protein activity. Several compounds that alter membrane-lipid properties can activate various protein kinases such as PKC, PKA and MAPKs involved in the stress response.

Also, a direct drug-protein interaction is not necessarily required for changes in membrane lipids to alter membrane protein activity. Thus, modification of membrane properties is required to change specific mechanisms such as the signaling pathways that alter/induce HSP expression.

A restructuring of microdomain organization of membranes is influenced by subtle alterations of membrane lipids and has therapeutic potentials in heart ailments, in which HSP and membrane-property dysregulation occur simultaneously reflecting a common signaling cascade controlled by membrane hyperstructures and affects HSP expression.

Therefore, it has been proposed by Vigh and co-workers (2007) that membrane lipids are vital for proper cell signaling and for HSP expression and function.

5.5. HSPs in Vaccine Development

HSPs possess many functional roles, however, their intrinsic ability to stimulate innate and antigen-specific immunity have made them attractive candidates in vaccine development. Beachy and colleagues have reported in Methods (2007) the use of genetically engineered molecular chaperones to promote anti-tumor responses suggesting the interplay of HSPs in cell-based vaccine development. There have been earlier reports on the development of recombinant HSP110-HER-2/*neu* vaccine using the chaperoning properties of HSP110 for tumor suppression because of the ability of HSPs to bind tumor-specific peptides. This is also true if we extrapolate the potency of HSPs as vaccines in CVDs. This is a promising approach towards treatment of vascular disorders in a new facet of HSP therapy.

References

Beachy SH, Kisailus AJ, Repasky EA, Subjeck JR, Wang XY and Kazim AL (2007) Engineering secretable forms of chaperones for immune modulation and vaccine development. *Methods* 43: 184-193.

Brundel BJJM, Ke L, Dijkhuis AJ, Qi XY, Takeshita AS, Nattel S, Henning RH and Kampinga HH (2008) Heat shock proteins as molecular targets for intervention in atrial fibrillation. *Cardiovasc. Res.* 78: 422-428.

Griffin TM, Valdez T and Mestril R (2004) Radicicol activates heat shock protein expression and cardioprotection in neonatal rat cardiomyocytes. *Am. J. Physiol. Heart Circ. Physiol.* 287: H1081-H1088.

Latchman DS (2001) Heat shock proteins and cardiac protection. *Cardiovasc. Res.* 51: 637-646.

Melo LG, PachoriAS, Gnecchi M and Dzau VJ (2005) Genetic therapies for cardiovascular diseases. *Trends Mol. Med.* 11: 240-250.

Vign L, Horvath I, Maresca B and Harwood JL (2007) Can the stress protein response be controlled by 'membrane-lipid therapy'?.*Trends Biochem. Sci.* 32: 357-363.

Index

P

Q